Controlling Hospital Costs

MIT Press Series in Health and Public Policy
Jeffrey E. Harris, general editor

1. *Professionalism and the Public Interest: Price and Quality in Optometry,*
James W. Begun, 1981.

2. *Controlling Hospital Costs: The Role of Government Regulation,*
Paul L. Joskow, 1981.

3. *Biomedical Innovation,* edited by Edward B. Roberts, Robert I. Levy,
Stan N. Finkelstein, Jay Moskowitz, and Edward J. Sondik, 1981.

4. *An Ounce of Prevention: Child Health Politics under Medicaid,*
Anne-Marie Foltz, 1982.

Controlling Hospital Costs

The Role of Government Regulation

Paul L. Joskow

The MIT Press
Cambridge, Massachusetts, and London, England

First paperback printing, 1984

This book was set in Palatino by Grafacon, Inc. and printed and
bound by Halliday Lithograph in the United States of America.

Library of Congress Cataloging in Publication Data

Joskow, Paul L.
  Controlling hospital costs.

  (MIT Press series in health and public policy; 2)
  Bibliography: p.
  Includes index.
  1. Hospitals—United States—Cost control. 2. Hospitals—Economic
aspects—United States. 3. Hospitals—Cost control—Law and legislation—
United States. I. Title. II. Series. [DNLM: 1. Cost control. 2. Economics,
Hospital—United States. 3. Government—United States. 4. Health
policy—United States. 5. Insurance, Health—United States. W1 MI938 v.
2 / WX 157 J83c]
RA981.A2J65   362.1'1'0681   81-14289
ISBN 0-262-60012-9   AACR2

for Barbara

Contents

Series Foreword

This M.I.T. Press series serves as a forum for significant new research in the field of health and public policy. The series encompasses current problems in health-care organization, financing, and regulation. It also focuses on emerging policy problems in environmental health, workplace safety, toxic substances, and the assessment of new medical technology. We plan to publish original scholarly monographs, highly focused collections by multiple authors, and textbooks that explore new fields.

In this volume Paul L. Joskow of the Massachusetts Institute of Technology, a distinguished contributor to the economics of government regulation, analyzes regulatory controls on hospital costs. The book sets out a general framework for evaluating government interventions in the hospital sector. Within this framework, Joskow examines the United States experience with controls on hospital capital expenditures and the regulation of hospital reimbursement. He concludes with an overall assessment of government regulation as a long-run strategy for controlling hospital costs in this country. The author has made a major contribution to the continuing public-policy debate on the role of the state in the market for hospital services.

Jeffrey E. Harris

Acknowledgments

This book is based on research conducted over a three-year period and focused on hospital economics and the prospects and problems of economic regulation applied to the hospital sector. The research has been financed by grants from the National Science Foundation (SOC78-02014) and the Sloan Foundation. Additional support was provided by the Department of Economics at the Massachusetts Institute of Technology and the John F. Kennedy School of Government at Harvard, where I was a visiting professor during the 1979–1980 academic year. While preparing this book and several related papers, I have been fortunate to have had the assistance of Reed Shuldiner, Michael Salinger, Mark Levonian, and George Pennacchi.

As this research has proceeded, I have benefited greatly from comments, suggestions, and discussions with numerous colleagues. I would like to thank Jeffrey Harris, Richard Schmalensee, Charles Phelps, Joseph Newhouse, Peter Temin, Christopher DeMuth, Richard Zechauser, and Mark Pauly for their helpful comments. Mancur Olson and Robert Helms provided helpful comments and encouragement on an earlier version of this material, which I presented at a conference sponsored by the American Enterprise Institute. A shorter version of several chapters of this book has been published as "Alternative Regulatory Mechanism for Controlling Hospital Costs," in the conference volume edited by Mancur Olson: *Health Care—Professional Ethics, Government Regulation, or Markets?*, American Enterprise Institute, Washington, D.C. 1981. I am especially grateful to William B. Schwartz, who aroused my interest in this subject and with whom I have collaborated on several papers.

Acknowledgments

Controlling Hospital Costs

Hospital Costs and Government Regulation

By almost any criterion the provision of hospital care in the United States is big business. Expenditures in community hospitals now amount to about $80 billion dollars per year and account for an increasing share of national income. Including physician's fees, the costs incurred by hospital patients amount to nearly $100 billion per year. Over 35 million patients are treated on an inpatient basis each year, and community hospitals provided care on an outpatient basis to over 200 million patients. Over 2½ million nurses, technicians, orderlies, and administrative personnel are employed by community hospitals, and about 400,000 physicians rely on hospitals to care for their patients. Most communities pride themselves on the quality and sophistication of their hospital care. As a nation we like to think that the highest quality medical and hospital care possible is available to us. Along with most developed countries, the United States has gone a long way to ensure that this care is available to all without regard to income, age, sex, or race.

Yet all is not well in our community hospital system. The rapid increase in the availability and sophistication of diagnostic and therapeutic services in American hospitals has made them increasingly expensive. We have all borne these costs in one way or another. Premiums for private hospital insurance coverage have increased in lockstep with the costs of hospital care and represent a growing share of business expenses and individual disposable income. The two major public hospital insurance programs, Medicare and Medicaid, designed to provide hospital care at low out-of-pocket costs to the elderly, the disabled, and the indigent, have been placing an increasingly painful burden on federal and state budgets, which are hard pressed to pay for existing programs while responding to public demands for reduced taxes. These programs have become major contributors to the "uncontrollable" expenses of local, state, and federal government.

The rapid increases in hospital expenditures, the general concern with inflationary forces in the economy, the fiscal pressures faced by all levels of government, and the desire by many to save the benefits of the Medicare and Medicaid programs from the budget cutters' scalpels necessarily raise serious questions about our hospital system. Is what the hospital system providing worth the cost of the scarce resources that it is consuming? Can major changes in the way hospital care is provided and payed for yield approximately equivalent levels of care less expensively? Many analysis believe that the answer to the first question is no and that the answer to the second question is yes. This conclusion has, in turn, led many, especially those in government, to favor a variety of administrative schemes for regulating the supply and demand for hospital services with the objective of reducing public and private expenditures for hospital care.

Until the late 1960s most government interventions in the hospital sector were oriented toward improving the availability and quality of hospital services. The Hill-Burton program provided federal funds and subsidized loans to build additional hospital facilities and to modernize existing facilities. There was a substantial commitment to financing research and development activities designed to increase our understanding of the causes of illness and disease and to develop new diagnostic and therapeutic techniques for improving the quality of care. Planning agencies were created to help ensure that needed facilities were built in a timely manner. A plethora of rules and regulations were promulgated to help ensure that only well-qualified personnel treated patients in safe, well-maintained, and up-to-date facilities. The federal income tax system provided substantial subsidies to offset partially the costs of private insurance purchases. The Medicare and Medicaid programs were initiated to provide health and hospital insurance to the elderly, the disabled, and the poor. Public hospitals were built and expanded by state and local governments to care for those who could not obtain care elsewhere. At least since the Second World War, government has played a pervasive role in expanding both the demand for and the supply of hospital care. With minor exceptions, however, the government did not play the role of economic regulator in the hospital sector as it did in transportation, energy, and telecommunications. Indeed, leading texts and treatises on economic regulation do not even mention the hospital system or health care. It has not traditionally been considered a regulated industry.

This orientation has changed over the past ten years. Both federal and state governments have shown greater concern with the costs of hospital care and have created administrative agencies empowered to control hospital costs. An extensive system of hospital facility planning and regulation has been promoted by the federal government, and numerous planning and certificate-of-need agencies have been created at the state and local levels in response to these federal initiatives. While these agencies retain statutory responsibilities to promote high-quality hospital care, they are also responsible for controlling costs and for eliminating waste and inefficiency. Several states have created rate-setting commissions to regulate hospital charges and the terms of reimbursement between hospitals and third-party payers. The Carter administration made a serious but unsuccessful effort to create a federal reimbursement regulation program. During the same time in which successful efforts were made to reduce the power of government agencies to regulate supply, demand, and prices in many sectors of the economy, the trend in the hospital sector has been just the reverse. More extensive economic regulation is seen by some as the only feasible means for reducing hospital expenditures and for eliminating perceived waste and inefficiency.

Our experience with economic regulation in the traditional regulated sectors, shows that effective regulation in the public interest is often difficult to achieve. Unregulated markets may yield less than ideal results, and a theoretical rationale for some form of economic regulation in these cases can often be developed. Even in the best of circumstances, however, regulatory agencies have been able to deal only imperfectly with the perceived problems. In many cases regulation has been able to alleviate some market allocation problems only at the expense of creating others. In the worst cases regulation has not solved the problems that its early advocates sought to address while it simultaneously created other distortions that have been costly to consumers, producers or both. The shortcomings of economic regulation are attributable partly to difficult technical problems associated with efforts to control consumer and producer behavior with a limited array of instruments and imperfect information. However, the political and legal environment frequently has profound implications for the regulatory process and its outcomes.

Although the effectiveness and desirability of government regulation in particular situations is disputed, there are also many areas of broad agreement. Four such areas are of particular importance in evaluating alternative forms of economic regulation of the hospital system. First, before creating administrative agencies to deal with perceived problems of resource misallocation in any industry, we must understand the allocation of resources in that industry and the structural and behavioral factors that lead to poor industry performance. Second, the empirical consequence of perceived performance failures must be large enough to justify the creation of a costly and necessarily imperfect administrative process. At best, rolling out the regulatory artillery is likely to pay only if it will be shooting at large targets. Third, a wide array of administrative approaches and regulatory instruments are likely to be feasible for dealing with poor economic performance, some much more productive than others. In choosing among them, we must try to tie the regulatory intervention to the causes of the poor performance, not just to their symptoms. Great care must be taken to evaluate the information required to implement strategies and the administrative costs of alternative strategies. It is also important to understand the ways in which consumers and producers can respond and adapt regulatory instruments, since countervailing actions by regulated agents can frequently lead to outcomes that are even more costly than the original problems regulation sought to address. Fourth, we must not forget that any regulatory system operates in the context of a complex political process and is subject to the legal constraints of the Constitution and federal and state administrative law. In short, we must think twice before moving forward with economic regulation and, if we move forward, work hard to define an effective regulatory process.

In light of the extensive interest in regulating the hospital sector and the diverse and often disappointing results of government regulation in other sectors, a complete theoretical and empirical analysis of economic regulation of hospitals seems useful. This book is an effort to provide such an analysis. It draws on the theoretical and empirical tools of economics and the application of these tools to issues of government regulation. I do not intend this study to be the last word on government regulation applied to hospitals. However, I do hope that it provides a comprehensive theoretical and empirical economic framework for evaluating alternative regulatory instruments and for guiding future applications of economic regulation in this sector.

I offer no easy solutions. Instead I paint a gloomy picture of the long-run value of several of the regulatory programs that have been advanced. There appear to be severe problems of resource misallocation to and within the hospital system. But many of the proposed regulatory solutions are poorly suited to deal with them effectively. The most promising regulatory instruments for dealing with the poor performance of the hospital sector raise difficult administrative, equity, and political problems. We cannot ignore fundamental conflicts between the national objective of providing the highest quality medical care possible, as perceived by patients and their physicians, without regard to ability to pay and the simultaneous objective of reducing the resources devoted to providing that care. There are no easy solutions to these problems, whether regulatory of nonregulatory, and I suggest that certain forms of government regulation that apply modest general budget constraints to hospitals are better than the status quo and may provide useful short-run improvements in the allocation of resources. These forms of government regulation may be useful transitional devices for controlling hospital costs as our society pursues more fundamental changes in the delivery of hospital care, the payment of hospital insurance, and the ways in which individuals and society make decisions about the kinds of care they want.

The Economic Characteristics of the American Hospital System

To understand the motivations for government regulation of hospital costs and the prospects and problems associated with regulatory alternatives, we must first develop a complete picture of the economic characteristics of the hospital system: the structure of the hospital system, the nature of hospital utilization, the costs of providing hospital care, the financing of hospital care, and the changes in these characteristics over time.

Number, Size, and Service Distribution

Today there are about 6,000 acute-care hospitals (excluding federal hospitals) operating in the United States (table 2.1).[1] These hospitals are predominantly nonprofit institutions. About 60 percent are private, nonprofit organizations established under either secular or religious auspices. Another 30 percent are hospitals owned by state and local governments. Only about 10 percent are private for-profit institutions. Its predominantly non-profit character distinguishes the American hospital system from other industries that have been subject to extensive economic regulation.[2] It also has important implications for the goals that hospitals are thought to pursue and the command and control system that determines the allocation of resources within hospitals.

The 6,000 acute-care hospitals contain almost 1 million beds, provide varied inpatient and outpatient services, have treated over 35 million inpatients and 200 million outpatients, and have accumulated about $66 billion in expenditures (excluding physicians fees), or about 2.8 percent of the gross national product (GNP) in 1979. However, there is no simple characterization that can reasonably define a "typical" hospital. Indeed, an important characteristic of this sector is the tremendous diversity among hospitals. Consider size (table 2.1). Community hospitals vary from fewer than 25 beds to over 1,000 beds. Nearly half of the hospitals have fewer than 100 beds while less than 30 percent have more than 200 beds. However, the relatively small fraction of hospitals with 200 beds or more provide most of the care and incur most of the expenditures. These hospitals treat nearly 70 percent of all

Table 2.1 Distribution of Short-Term Hospitals by Ownership and Size, 1979

Type of Ownership Bed-Size Category	Number of Hospitals	Number of Beds	Number of Admissions (millions)	Expenditures ($ billions)
Nongovernment/ nonprofit	3,350	690,000	24.9	48
Investor-owned/ for profit	727	83,000	3.0	5
State/local government	1,846	214,000	7.3	13
Total	5,923	988,000	35.2	66
6–24	292	5,553	0.2	0.2
25–49	1,090	39,545	1.3	1.5
50–99	1,463	104,992	3.6	4.7
100–199	1,385	195,401	7.0	10.9
200–299	718	173,273	6.5	11.4
300–399	402	135,939	5.1	9.9
400–499	251	110,825	4.1	8.7
500+	322	222,159	7.4	18.9

Source: *Hospital Statistics 1980.* Chicago: American Hospital Association, 1980.

inpatients and account for about 75 percent of all community hospital expenditures. The vast majority of teaching hospitals and hospitals affiliated with medical schools are in the largest size categories.

Hospitals differ in much more than bed capacity. There are also enormous differences in the kinds of services provided. All hospitals offer basic nursing care and have facilities for performing simple X rays and surgical procedures, but less than a third have premature nurseries, fewer than 20 percent have hemodialysis units, 10 percent have open-heart surgery facilities, 20 percent have computed tomography (CT) scanners, and 3 percent have organ banks.[3] Less than 20 percent of the hospitals have approved residency programs of any type, and a small percentage have full-time house staff physicians. The larger hospitals are more likely than the smaller hospitals to offer a complete range of diagnostic and therapeutic services, to treat more complicated medical problems, and to incur greater expenses. As a result, in formulating public policies for the hospital sector, we must recognize that the grouping of an extremely diverse set of institutions into the general category short-term hospitals is only a matter of convenience.

There are also significant regional differences in the supply of hospital beds and facilities. The number of beds per capita varies from about 5.7 per thousand in the West North Central region to 3.7 per thousand in the Mountain region. The number of personnel per bed varies from 3.2 in New England to about 2.3 in the West North Central region. The average cost per hospital stay varies from $1,950 in New England and the Middle Atlantic region to about $1,200 in the East South Central region.[4] The most sophisticated diagnostic and therapeutic services are more likely to be located in urban areas in the Northeast, Midwest, and Pacific regions than in rural areas or the South. Urban residents are likely to live near several hospitals offering different types of care, while rural residents often have to travel long distances to obtain access to a similar array of services.

Utilization, Costs, and Methods of Payment

In 1979 community hospitals incurred expenditures of about $66 billion exclusive of physician's fees. (Total hospital expenditures including federal hospitals and long-term care facilities amounted to over $85 billion.) About 88 percent of these expenditures were for inpatient care, about 12 percent for outpatient care. This implies inpatient expenditures of about $215 per day and about $1,600 per admission. Outpatient care cost about $40 per visit.

Hospital utilization also varies considerably by age group. Older individuals are more likely than younger individuals to be hospitalized (table 2.2) and are more likely to require inpatient care for longer periods of time. People over 65 account for over a third of the inpatient days of care even though this age group accounts for only about 10 percent of the population. About 40 percent of those hospitalized undergo at least one surgical procedure.

Hospitalization rates vary by region, from about 140 per thousand in the Pacific to a high of about 185 per thousand in the East South Central region. There are also significant regional differences in the average legnth of stay. For example, the average length of stay in the Middle Atlantic is 9 days, but only 6.5 days in the Pacific region. Neither the differences in hospitalization rates nor the differences in average length of stay can be fully explained by regional differences in the age distribution of the

Table 2.2 Hospital Utilization by Age, 1978

Age Group (years)	Civilian Population (percent)	Discharges (percent)	Days of Care (percent)	Average Stay (days)	Surgery (percent)
<15	23.7	9.8	5.9	4.4	41.8
15–44	45.3	42.2	30.5	5.3	46.1
45–64	20.3	23.5	27.2	8.5	42.0
65+	10.7	24.4	36.4	11.0	31.8

Source: *Utilization of Short-Stay Hospitals—1978*. Washington, D.C. Department of Health, Education, and Welfare, March 1980. DHEW Publication No. (PHS) 80-1797.

Table 2.3 Hospital Utilization by Length of Stay, 1978

Length of Stay (days)	Percentage of Discharges
<1	2.8
1	8.3
2	15.1
3	13.2
4	10.6
5–6	14.5
7–8	10.0
9–10	6.6
11–20	13.1
21–30	3.4
31+	2.4

Source: *Utilization of Short-Stay Hospitals—1978*. Washington, D.C.: Department of Health, Education, and Welfare, March 1980. DHEW Publication No. (PHS) 80-1797.

population.[5] Since patients admitted to hospitals have a wide variety of medical problems, the time they spend in the hospital and the resources expended in caring for them vary enormously from individual to individual. About half of the inpatients spend 4 or fewer days in the hospital, while about 20 percent of the patients stay in the hospital for more than 10 days (table 2.3).

One of the most important characteristics of the hospital sector is the way that this care is paid for. Unlike most other sectors of the economy, the typical patient pays directly for only a tiny fraction of the cost of the services that he consumes (table 2.4). Most of the population has some form of hospital insurance, which

Table 2.4 Expenditures on Hospital Care and Sources of Payment, 1950–1979 (in billions of dollars, percentages in parentheses)

Year	Total Expenditures	Direct Payments	Private Insurance	Public Insurance	Other
1950	3.9	1.1 (28)	0.7 (18)	1.9 (49)	0.1 (3)
1960	9.1	1.8 (20)	3.3 (36)	3.8 (42)	0.2 (2)
1965	13.9	2.4 (17)	5.8 (42)	6.9 (50)	0.3 (2)
1970	27.8	2.8 (10)	10.0 (36)	14.6 (53)	0.4 (1)
1975	52.1	4.0 (8)	18.8 (36)	28.9 (55)	0.5 (1)
1979	85.3	6.9 (8)	29.8 (35)	47.7 (56)	0.9 (1)

Source: Derived from data in *Health Care Financing Review,* Summer 1980, pp. 17–23. Department of Health, Education, and Welfare, Health Care Financing Administration (HCFA Publication No. 03054).

covers most of the charges incurred while a patient is in the hospital. For individuals under 65, reimbursement is generally provided under either a group or individual insurance plan purchased from Blue Cross or from a commercial insurer, usually a life insurance company. While coverage varies, these plans normally provide for a small deductible payment which the patient must pay. In addition, the patient may have to pay a small fraction of the charges for certain services provided in the hospital. Many individuals have insurance plans in which out-of-pocket expenditures are virtually zero.

Individuals over 65 are generally covered by public funds provided under the Medicare program and often have supplementary private coverage. Those enrolled in the Medicare program paid a deductible of $180 in 1980. Covered inpatient care is then fully reimbursed up to the sixtieth day. After 60 days Medicare patients are subject to a copayment requirement. Beyond 90 days Medicare allows patients to draw on a 60-day lifetime reserve which requires a higher copayment. Once the lifetime reserve is exhausted, Medicare coverage ends for longer stays. (Disabled persons and those with end-stage renal disease are also covered under the Medicare program.) Physician's fees and outpatient services are reimbursed under the supplementary insurance provisions with an annual deductible of $60 and a coinsurance rate of 20 percent. About 60 percent of those over 65 have some form of supplementary private insurance coverage to pay for all or part of the hospital costs not covered by Medicare.[6] On average, Medicare patients are liable for 6 percent of the hospital bill, most in the form of a deductible.

This excludes supplementary private coverage.

Low-income individuals satisfying federal and state eligibility requirements are covered for hospital expenditures under the Medicaid program, the costs of which are shared by the federal government and the states. The federal government has established minimum eligibility and coverage requirements, which the states must adhere to as participants in the program. Beyond the federal minimum requirements, both eligibility and coverage vary considerably from state to state. The extent to which the poverty population is covered by Medicaid and other public assistance programs is not well documented, but the coverage is far from complete.[7]

In the aggregate (table 2.4) direct payments by patients, exclusive of insurance premiums, account for less than 10 percent of hospital expenditures. Private insurance plans account for about 35 percent of hospital expenditures, and public programs financed by federal and state governments account for about 55 percent of hospital expenditures. Over the past 30 years direct payments by individuals have increased by a factor of 7, while payments by state and federal governments have increased by a factor of 25. Although the precise levels of coverage of the various private and public programs are not known, it appears that between 80 percent and 90 percent of the population has fairly extensive hospital insurance coverage. In a recent survey of anticipated sources of payment, only about 5 percent of the patients expected that they rather than some public or private program would be the major source of payment for hospitalization (table 2.5). The typical insured patient probably pays about 5 percent of the hospital charges incurred.

That such a large proportion of the population has extensive insurance coverage for hospitalization has profound implications for the demand for hospital care and the changes that have occurred in costs and utilization over the past 20 years. The methods by which third-party payers reimburse hospitals also have important implications for the incentives of hospitals to provide various levels of care and to do so efficiently.

Changes in Expenditures and Utilization
The hospital sector of today is far different from the hospital sector that existed 10 or 20 years ago, in terms of real resource costs and

Table 2.5 Distribution of Expected Principal Sources of Payment for
Patients Discharged from Short-Stay Hospitals, 1977

Source of Payment	Percentage of Discharges	Average Length of Stay (days)
Private Insurance	44.1	6.0
Workmen's Compensation	1.8	7.3
Medicare	38.2	10.9
Medicaid	7.3	6.6
Other Government	2.5	6.1
Self-Pay	4.6	5.2
No Charge	0.2	6.8
Other	1.2	6.4

Source: *Expected Principal Source of Payment for Hospital Discharges; United States,
1977.* Advance data, U.S. Department of Health and Human Services, Office of
Health Research, Statistics, and Technology, Number 62, October 31, 1980.

in terms of the quantities and types of care that it provides. The
American hospital system has been changing rapidly along almost
every dimension. Indeed, these dramatic changes, especially the
growth in real resources going to hospital care, have been a prime
motivation for government regulation. Those who defend the current system point proudly to the large increases in the inpatient
and outpatient utilization of hospitals and the dramatic changes
in the kinds of therapeutic and diagnostic services now available,
at negligible out-of-pocket cost, to almost the entire population.
Detractors point to the enormous growth in expenditures and the
increasing costs of public and private health insurance as indicative
of a wasteful and inefficient system that must be controlled by
government fiat.

Table 2.6 presents aggregate U.S. data on indicators of hospital
expenditures and utilization for the last two decades. Over this
time, real hospital expenditures have increased at a compound
annual rate of about 9.5 percent per year,[8] but the real rate of
growth in expenditures fluctuated considerably. It was highest
during the 1966–1970 period, following the introduction of Medicare and Medicaid, declined during the first five years of this
decade, and has continued to decline to date. Real expenditure
increases over the past five years are lower, perhaps substantially
lower,[9] than they were in the five years preceding the introduction

Table 2.6 Hospital Expenditures and Hospital Utilization, Nonfederal Short-Term Hospitals (compound rates of growth)

	1960–1979	1960–1966	1966–1970	1970–1975	1975–1979
Expenditures	13.9	10.7	17.5	14.8	14.1
Hospitals	0.5	1.2	0.2	0.4	0.2
Beds	2.3	3.1	2.5	2.2	1.1
Admissions	2.3	2.7	2.1	2.8	1.2
Adjusted Patient-Days	NA	NA	3.0	2.1	1.1
Average Cost per Stay	NA	NA	15.1	11.1	12.3
Consumer Price Index	5.0	1.5	4.6	6.7	8.5
GNP Deflator	4.8	1.9	4.4	6.8	7.1
Hospital Input Price Index (HCFA)	NA	NA	NA	7.8	8.8
Hospital Input Price Index (AHA)	NA	NA	NA	7.1	9.0

Source: Derived from American Hospital Association data and federal government data (various years).

of Medicare and Medicaid. Qualitatively identical patterns of expenditure growth characterize the regions of the country.

It is useful to think of hospital expenditures as being composed of three basic components: (1) changes in the cost of inputs (labor, capital, materials); (2) changes in the quantity of services provided, reflecting population growth, changes in the demographic characteristics of the population (especially the age distribution), and changes in individual demands for care resulting from increases in real incomes and changes in insurance coverage; and (3) changes in the scope of services offered by the hospital sector, reflecting both technological change and changes in the demand for hospital services.

We can imagine a static world in which input prices are fixed, per capita incomes are constant, and there is no technological change. In this case we would expect population growth to lead to increasing hospital utilization and increasing hospital expenditures which "replicate" what is being provided to the existing population. The cost per day or per hospital stay would not change. Next we can consider factors that increase the typical individual's demand for hospital care, factors such as increases in per capita income, reductions in the net price of hospital care associated with more extensive insurance coverage, life-style and environmental factors affecting health status, and changing perceptions about the value of hospital care. Increases in demand imply that patients are willing to pay for more and better care given the existing opportunity set for providing hospital care. By allowing individual demands to increase, even holding the population constant, we would expect to see additional hospital admissions and increases in the services provided. Expenditures on hospital care would increase as the increased demands are satisfied. These increases would show up as increases in hospital admissions and increases in the intensity of care provided to hospitalized individuals—more diagnostic tests, better nursing care, and more treatments provided per hospital stay—increasing the expenditures per hospital admission.

We can also imagine the effects of new and improved diagnostic and therapeutic modalities. The new modalities have value to patients; when the new services become available, they want these services to be provided. Additional expenditures are incurred as the new services are provided to the population. The intensity of care, in terms of resource expenditures per capita, per admission, or per day of care, increases as a result of new therapeutic and diagnostic techniques. New equipment must be purchased, and additional personnel must be hired. As the costs of inputs rise, we would expect the costs of hospital care to rise as well, reflecting the increased payments for nurses, equipment, and supplies.

The hospital sector over the past 20 years has been characterized by changes in all these dimensions. The population has been growing, per capita income has been rising, insurance coverage has been improving, and the state of medical technology has changed rapidly. Thus it should not be surprising that expenditures on hospital care have also been increasing continuously over the past 20 years, measured in any way one chooses.

Table 2.7 presents two indexes for hospital input prices and a third index (HII), which measures the changes in real resource inputs per inpatient day. The cost of hospital inputs has been rising somewhat faster than the general rate of inflation in the economy. More important, real resource inputs per inpatient day have been rising at a rate of about 4.5 percent per year. Thus the intensity of care has been increasing very rapidly.[10] Taken together

Table 2.7 Hospital Input Cost Indexes and Hospital Intensity Index (annual rates of change—%)

	Hospital Cost Index (HCI)	Hospital Input Price Index (HIPI)	Hospital Intensity Index (HII)
1970	8.7	7.5	9.6
1971	6.3	6.4	5.3
1972	3.4	5.8	3.2
1973	4.9	6.0	1.8
1974	9.2	10.1	4.0
1975	11.9	10.6	4.6
1976	10.3	8.8	5.8
1977	9.1	8.1	4.4
1978	7.2	8.4	4.8
1979	9.3	10.1	2.8

Source: Derived from American Hospital Association (HCI and HII) and Health Care Financing Administration (HIPI) data.

with the data in table 2.6, these data show that about 60 percent of the increase in expenditures results from increases in input prices (which may be partially induced by other factors). About 10 percent results from additional admissions and outpatient visits (reflecting population growth and increases in individual demands for care). Finally, about 30 percent results from increases in the intensity of care. Input price changes aside, about 75 percent of the increase in real resource expenditures is the result of increases in the quantity, quality, and scope of services provided.

If the hospital sector were characterized by static technology, it might be surprising that the intensity of care could increase at such a rapid rate for so long and still confer additional benefits to patients. The available diagnostic and therapeutic techniques, however, are constantly changing. This rapid technological change can occur in two dimensions. First, new ways of providing existing diagnostic and therapeutic services may be found, reducing the cost of providing these services (process innovations).[11] Second, new diagnostic and therapeutic services that can improve health care outcomes may become available (product innovations). Product innovations may supplement or replace existing services and may be more or less expensive than the services they replace.

Technological change over the past two decades has been heavily weighted toward product rather than process innovations, toward innovations that supplement rather than replace existing diagnostic modalities, and toward more expensive rather than less expensive techniques.[12] As a result, technological change is viewed by some policymakers as a major cause of a serious cost problem, and unlike technological change in any other industry, technological change in the hospital sector is often regarded as bad by those concerned with cost containment.

The relationship between innovation and costs depends on the nature of the process that determines the rate and direction of technological change and the ways in which new technologies are utilized. A general perception is that a significant fraction of increased hospital expenditures results from the application of diagnostic and therapeutic techniques that were not available 10 or 20 years ago. However, no one can hope to estimate this fraction with any precision given the aggregate data on capital, labor, and materials inputs that are commonly used in the analysis of hospital costs.

More disaggregated data provide additional evidence that more intensive use of newer diagnostic and therapeutic techniques accounts for a significant portion of the increase in real resources devoted to hospital care. Table 2.8 presents data for median "small" and "large" hospitals on the annual rate of growth of the revenues derived from a large number of profit centers in these hospitals over the period 1972–1976.[13] Post-1976 data are not presented in exactly the same form, but the general trends indicated appear to have continued at least through 1978.

Of most interest are the differential growth rates in expenditures observed for the various service centers of the hospital. The largest increases in inpatient expenditures are associated with intensive care units, intravenous therapy, inhalation therapy, and central services and supply—areas in which expenditures for many new diagnostic and therapeutic techniques are likely to appear. Inpatient expenditures for anesthesiology, pharmacy, laboratory, and radiology (for smaller hospitals) have tended to increase at a rate somewhat below the general rate of increase in expenditures.

Expenditures on basic medical, surgical, and obstetrical nursing units (the "beds") have increased at rates substantially below those for ancillary services and for the hospital as a whole. These data are inconsistent with much of the rhetoric concerning the sources of increasing hospital expenditures. Proponents of economic regulation appear to be preoccupied with changes in the number of

Table 2.8 Estimated Increases in Expenditures (annual percentage change 1972–1976)

Service	>400 Beds	100–149 Beds
Medical, Surgical Nursing	10.4	8.9
Obstetrical Suite	12.4	11.4
Operating and Recovery Rooms	16.7	16.4
Laboratory, Inpatient	13.7	13.5
Radiology, Inpatient	15.2	13.3
Blood Bank	16.8	19.9
Pharmacy	13.6	11.8
Anesthesiology	12.0	12.5
Intensive and Coronary Care	19.6	20.4
Intravenous Therapy	19.0	23.2
Inhalation Therapy	17.7	18.0
Central Services and Supply	19.6	18.2
Emergency Services	16.4	24.1
Laboratory, Outpatient	21.1	21.6
Radiology, Outpatient	21.4	18.6
Clinics	18.5	35.4
Physical Therapy	19.9	20.6
Other Patient Care	22.5	22.1

Source: Derived from data collected by the Hospital Administrative Service of the American Hospital Association (various years).

hospital beds and occupancy rates. These data indicate that it is not the "beds" that are important but what is done for patients once they occupy those beds.

Finally, outpatient expenditures have been increasing at a much faster rate than inpatient expenditures. This trend reflects the increasingly important role that hospitals play in providing ambulatory services, the increasing availability and sophistication of emergency services, and, perhaps, a substituion of outpatient care for inpatient care.

Another way to quantify the rate and direction of technological change is to make time-series comparisons of the number of hospitals offering particular services. As new technologies are developed, we expect to observe them diffusing over time to a larger number of hospitals and to be able to measure the spread of new technology by counting the number of hospitals offering particular services. (This exercise is largely structured by the way that the American Hospital Association collects this kind of data.) Table 2.9 provides some examples of this procedure by comparing the number of hospitals with eight diagnostic and therapeutic services associated with improvements in quality and increases in intensity in 1972 and 1979. Many more hospitals were offering these services in 1979 than in 1972, but merely determining whether a hospital has an intensive care unit does not tell us much about its size, equipment, or personnel. Most hospitals have clinical laboratories, but the equipment for performing lab tests has changed. Many hospitals have diagnostic radioisotope facilities, but not all have CT scanners.[14] The availability of the equipment and personnel necessary to perform open-heart surgery tells us little about the number of surgeons trained to perform such surgery or advances in technique that allow this procedure to be made available to a larger number of patients. (Between 1972 and 1979 the number of open-heart procedures increased by a factor of three or four.)[15] In short, this count gives us only a rough picture of the spread of new medical technology. It almost certainly underestimates the rate of technological change.

The number of hospitals in the United States has not changed much over the past ten years. Bed capacity has increased with the growth in the average size of the typical community hospital. More important, however, the range of medical services available

Table 2.9 Short-Term Hospitals Offering Particular Services

	1972	1979
Hospitals Reporting	5,456	5,319
Open-Heart Surgery	450	549
Histopathology Laboratory	2,611	2,960
Inhalation Therapy	3,556	4,675
Electro-encephalography	1,979	3,048
Hemodialysis	588	1,027
Genetic Counseling	154	290
Intensive Care (Cardiac Only)	1,924	1,660
Intensive Care (Mixed)	3,191	3,616

Source: *Hospital Statistics 1972* and *Hospital Statistics 1980.* American Hospital Association, Chicago, Ill.

in the smaller community hospitals has increased substantially over the past two decades. As the stock of medical specialists has increased, more specialists have come to practice in community hospitals outside the traditional tertiary care facilities located in medical teaching centers. Hospitals have competed for these specialists by providing more sophisticated diagnostic and therapeutic facilities, thus leading to greater dispersion of these facilities than existed two decades ago.[16] This diffusion may be slowing down, as many types of facilities have become almost fully saturated.

Conclusions

The hospital sector is diverse in terms of size, costs, kinds of services offered, and types of patients treated. It has been a very dynamic sector, in terms of the number of patients treated and the kinds of services offered. The costs of hospital care have increased quite rapidly as a result of increases in input prices, growth in the population, and changes in its composition. Most important, the nature of the product provided has changed enormously as the intensity of hospital care has increased in response to technological change and increases in the demand for hospital services. However, there is considerable evidence that the real rate of growth in hospital expenditures has been declining fairly steadily over the past ten years, especially in the past four or five years. The typical patient now pays only a very small proportion of the costs incurred directly, because most of the population now has extensive insurance coverage. The high and rapidly increasing real costs of hospital care have become a major source of public policy concern as private insurance premiums increase and government outlays grow.

3 Resource Allocation and the Performance of the Unregulated Market

The discussion in the previous chapter was descriptive rather than normative and leads immediately to a number of important questions that lie at the heart of the arguments for economic regulation of hospitals. Are the services being provided worth the costs? Are the services being supplied at the lowest cost possible? Does the interaction of a decentralized nonprofit hospital sector combined with extensive third-party, insurance coverage lead to waste and inefficiency? If the system is characterized by waste and inefficiency, what are the nature and the magnitude of the losses?

To answer these questions, I will examine the structural and behavioral characteristics of hospital demand, supply, and reimbursement policies that determine the allocation of resources to and within the hospital sector. The discussion draws extensively on theoretical and empirical work produced by health economists over the past ten years or so.

This theoretical discussion is useful for several reasons. First, recent discussions of hospital regulation implicitly assume that the hospital sector is characterized by enormous resource misallocations and that there is a resulting public interest rationale for government regulation.[1] This assumption is often justified by potentially misleading observations that hospital expenditures are increasing much faster than the general rate of inflation or that hospital expenditures consume a growing proportion of aggregate economic activity. These observations may be supplemented by a variety of crude ex post analyses comparing benefits and costs on the margin. However, I do not believe that these observations alone lead to useful quantitative or qualitative conclusions about the resource misallocation in the hospital sector or to the conclusion that administrative regulation provides a set of instruments that can improve the allocation of resources, considering all relevant factors.

Second, if the hospital sector is characterized by significant inefficiencies, the effective design of public policy instruments requires an understanding of the linkages between the structural and behavioral characteristics of this market and the poor performance. That is, we need to understand why prevailing market institutions perform poorly and the kinds of inefficiencies that particular institutional failures engender. Ideally, we would like to tie public policy solutions, whether administrative regulation or other public policies, to the causes of the problems, not just to the symptoms.

Research by economists and by other social scientists has generated a long list of potential market distortions, potential market imperfections, and related behavioral characteristics of patients, hospitals, and third-party payers. Such research has generally led to conclusions that we are paying much more for hospital care than it is worth.

The Role of Insurance

A great deal of the discussion concerning resource allocation problems in the hospital sector and in the health care system focuses on the extent of insurance coverage and the characteristics of insurance contracts. Since the need for and costs of health care are uncertain and since consumers are generally thought to be risk averse, the availability of at least some insurance will increase welfare by reducing uncertainty.[2] Once illness has occurred, however, the patient can choose among different levels of hospital care, each one using a different amount of resources as well as conferring potentially different expected benefits. The patient with some insurance has an ex post subsidy to the consumption of hospital care, which (ignoring transactions and monitoring costs) leads to an efficiency loss due to "moral hazard." The size of this loss depends on demand and supply conditions, including technological change, and on the opportunities to structure insurance contracts so as to deter inefficient consumption behavior by insured individuals when they become ill.

For example, assume that the expected cost of hospitalization is $2,000. If insured individuals have a coinsurance rate of 5 percent, then they can expect to pay only $100 if they become ill and seek hospital care. Consumption decisions are fully efficient only if care is provided to those patients who value that care at a level greater than or equal to $2,000. Since insured individuals face a price of only $100, care will be demanded if its value is greater than or equal to $100 rather than $2,000. If hospitals can supply all care demanded, "overconsumption" will result from the low out-of-pocket charges for hospital care, since some care supplied has a value less than the cost of supplying it. This is the nature of the efficiency loss due to moral hazard. The presence of this efficiency loss does not mean that insurance should not be made available. It means only that the risk-spreading benefits of insurance are at least partially offset by this type of overconsumption.

The optimal insurance contract, often characterized in theoretical models by an aggregate coinsurance rate, is determined by trading off the risk-spreading benefits of a lower coinsurance rate against the efficiency losses associated with the ex post subsidy on the consumption of care.[3] The more inelastic demand and supply are, the lower the optimal coinsurance will be, and vice versa. In the presence of moral hazard the optimal insurance contract will be incomplete in the sense that patients pay a fraction of the cost and have at least some incentive to restrict consumption. This insurance contract is optimal given assumptions about demand and supply responses.

To continue with the previous example, suppose that there were some way to costlessly screen patients so that only patients whose expected benefits exceed the expected costs actually gain admission; the rest are stopped at the door when they show up for care. Then there would be no moral hazard problem, and the optimal insurance contract would involve complete insurance. In this case supply is restricted by the screening mechanism, and some of those who might demand care because of the low coinsurance rate are not served. The costless screening assumption is obviously unrealistic, and hospitals have strong incentives under prevailing reimbursement arrangements to supply all care that is demanded, even if the expected value is low relative to the expected cost. At least with reference to some ideal insurance policy, the presence of moral hazard problems implies an inherent inefficiency in the hospital market. However, the system is inefficient only in relation to an abstract ideal, which is unlikely to be economically achievable. From a useful policy perspective, we can characterize the resulting allocation of resources as being inefficient only if we can identify institutional changes or government interventions that reduce the inefficiencies associated with moral hazard problems *without* incurring additional risk-bearing costs and transactions costs that exceed the implied savings.[4]

At one extreme, we can think of an insurance contract as promising to pay a fixed percentage of all costs incurred when the patient becomes ill, where the patient's consumption of health care is restricted only by the financial sacrifice imposed by the uniform coinsurance rate. We can also think of more complicated insurance contracts that seek to reduce moral hazard problems by restricting demand or supply responses. For example, a contract might have different coinsurance rates for different types of care or illnesses. Alternatively, fixed dollar payments for particular illnesses might be provided, representing an "appropriate" trade-off of the costs and benefits of care. At the other extreme, an insurance carrier could monitor the patient and cut off reimbursement when the quantity or quality of care exceeds some level. These contractual alternatives all represent methods for restricting either the demand for or the supply of care in particular situations. To the extent that such contractual improvements can be made costlessly, welfare will be improved. Unfortunately, transactions and monitoring costs appear to increase enormously as we try to write more restrictive contracts that maintain or increase risk-spreading benefits while reducing the extent of moral hazard.

It seems, therefore, that the moral hazard problem depends on more than individual demand elasticities. It is really a function of the ability and incentives that insurance firms have to write and enforce contracts that restrict ex post demand by patients or the supply responses of providers to reduce the associated inefficiencies. These factors in turn depend on information costs, monitoring costs, and the costs of writing insurance contracts tailored to individual preferences or hospital supply incentives. In a competitive insurance market we might expect these contracting costs to be taken into account, yielding optimal insurance contracts and an optimal amount of moral hazard.[5]

This leads to two observations. First, empirical studies determining that hospital resources are used to point where marginal benefits are less than marginal costs cannot in and of themselves imply that the market is performing inefficiently given the existence of moral hazard.[6] The "inefficiency" observed in this case would result from moral hazard, which by assumption cannot be economically reduced. Furthermore, the net welfare loss engendered by consuming too much care must be balanced on the margin by the risk-spreading benefits of the contract and the costs of writing and administering a more restrictive contract. Changing the contract to reduce the loss associated with moral hazard (by increasing coinsurance rates, for example) could be more than compensated for by the costs of increased risk bearing. Second, if moral hazard is the only source of inefficiency in the system (in some ideal sense), then regulatory efforts aimed at reducing it are likely to increase welfare only if they can somehow restrict demand and supply behavior more efficiently than the market can through prevailing insurance contracts between consumers and insurers or reimbursement arrangements between insurers and providers.

The assumption that insurance markets are competitive and that competitive insurance markets will yield optimal insurance contracts, given moral hazard, is the starting point for the literature that examines the resource-allocation effects of tax subsidies to health insurance premiums. The most extensive of these examinations have been conducted by Feldstein.[7] Feldstein observed that the U.S. tax system provides a major subsidy to the purchase of additional health insurance, since employer contributions for their employee's health insurance plans are tax-deductible business expenses but are not taxable income to the employee and are not included in the base on which Social Security taxes are levied. Feldstein and Friedman estimate that on the margin the subsidy amounts to about 35 percent of the premium. Mitchell and Phelps obtain similar results.[8] A subsidy that varies directly with the cost of the insurance purchased (in contrast to a lump sum subsidy) encourages individuals (presumably through their group plans) to purchase "too much" insurance, in the sense that coinsurance payments and deductibles will be lower than they would otherwise have been. Encouraging the purchase of more complete insurance increases ex post inefficiencies, reduces social welfare, and raises hospital expenditures. Feldstein imputes large welfare losses to these subsidies and argues that the prevalence of too much insurance is the major cause of the rapid rate of growth in the quantity, quality, and resource costs of hospital care.

In Feldstein's view the tax subsidies associated with employer contributions to group plans encourage consumers to purchase more complete insurance than they otherwise would. More complete insurance can be thought of as reducing the average coinsurance rate associated with group policies below what would represent the optimal trade-off between risk spreading and moral hazard. The net effect is to increase the efficiency loss associated with moral hazard by encouraging patients to consume larger amounts of hospital care. The cost of excessive insurance is rep-

resented by the incremental increases in the demand for and supply of hospital services compared with the demand and supply
responses associated with the optimal insurance package. The tax
subsidies do not cause the moral hazard problem; they simply
make it worse.

The view that there is too much insurance and the computations
that underlie estimates of the welfare losses and increases in hospital expenditures associated with this distortion do not necessarily
depend entirely on tax subsidies to the provision of private insurance. Only about half of the expenditures in acute hospitals
are attributable to patients with private insurance plans. The majority of hospital expenditures are paid for by government plans
(primarily Medicare and Medicaid) or by uninsured individuals.
To expand the notion that health insurance plans are generally
"too complete," there is a presumption that the federal and state
governments are providing too much insurance through the Medicare and Medicaid plans as well. The argument here is that the
coinsurance rates and deductibles that characterize the Medicare
program, for example, are too low or that government programs
do not otherwise monitor the consumption of care as well as they
could.

The importance of technological change in the hospital sector
may complicate this analysis considerably. Much of the literature
that allows for a dichotomy between quantity and quality of care
assumes that there is a fixed opportunity set of quantity-quality
combinations available at all times and from which any individual
consumer or patient can choose when determining insurance
coverage or the kinds of hospital care that he wants. Neither
assumption is appealing. The opportunity set of diagnostic and
therapeutic techniques is constantly changing.[9] How much of this
product innovation is exogenous and how much depends on the
completeness of insurance contracts is essentially unknown. Harris
has suggested that if the rate of technological change depends on
the aggregate coinsurance rate, we may face an externality problem
characterized by a failure of individuals to account properly for
the full social benefits of their insurance decisions as they affect
the development of valuable new services.[10] As a result, the private
market may yield too little insurance coverage. This view provides
support for at least some subsidies to the purchase of health
insurance. On the other hand, once technological change leads
to a range of new services that increase the opportunities for

higher quality care, the old, lower quality care may no longer be generally available.[11]

At any point in time the quality, sophistication, and costs of hospital care faced by any individual are functions of the demands placed on the system by all individuals. The large increases in Medicare and Medicaid benefits, for example, increased the demand for hospital services by the elderly and the poor. Simultaneously, the cost and quality of care generally available in the system increased as well. There is an interdependence between the demands placed on the system by individual groups of consumers and the supply characteristics of care available to all.[12] For example, the uninsured patient, who might prefer to choose from the "1960 set" of hospital care options, may find that the lower-cost and lower-quality components of that set are no longer available. This depends on two assumptions: first, that individual hospitals provide essentially one quality of care at any point in time and, second, that the hospital industry does not yield separate hospitals catering to the full range of consumer preferences. Both assumptions are quite plausible, and the availability of an opportunity set biased toward high-quality and high-cost bundles may actually encourage some consumers to purchase more complete insurance than they would otherwise want. The implication may thus be that the private market, even without subsidies, will yield too much insurance.

Despite these additional considerations, there seems to be a consensus among health economists that the hospital sector is characterized by excessive insurance, motivated by substantial tax incentives and government programs that provide overly extensive insurance.[13] Average, out-of-pocket expenditures on hospital care are less than 10 percent of total expenditures. The typical insured patient has an average coinsurance rate of about 5 percent, providing only a limited financial constraint on the demand for care.[14] The general view is that these insurance contracts are "too complete" and that excessive insurance coverage is the major cause of the welfare losses and leads to a level and rate of change in hospital expenditures that is "too high". Those who see this as the problem are attracted to solutions that eliminate the tax subsidies and change the terms of public insurance programs rather than resort to what Zeckhauser has called a "pyramiding of regulation"[15] in an attempt to cure one government-created distortion with a set of governmental controls that leaves the original distortion intact.

Although most of the literature has focused on the contractual relationships between consumers or patients and insurance companies, the nature of the contractual relationships between insurance firms and hospitals is also important. Third-party payers reimburse hospitals retrospectively, either according to the posted "charges" accumulated by a patient (up to the maximum in the insurance package less the coinsurance and deductible payments) or for the patient's "costs."[16] Private insurance firms and some Blue Cross plans pay the hospitals according to their posted charges (day rate, operating room charge, ancillary services). If one hospital has higher charges than another nearby hospital, the individual hospital's charges are reimbursed even if the patient could have obtained the same care more cheaply elsewhere. The majority of individuals covered by Blue Cross have contracts that reimburse a hospital for its "costs" as long as the costs are less than the charges. Costs were traditionally determined retrospectively based on the utilization of the hospital by typical patients, accounting conventions allocating costs to different types of care, and a reimbursement contract between Blue Cross and the individual hospital based on these computations.[17] Again, it is the individual hospital's costs that are relevant, whether they are higher or lower than those of other hospitals.

Medicare reimbursement and most Medicaid plans are also cost based in much the same way, although in the last few years reimbursement has become somewhat more restrictive.[18] Whether reimbursement is charge based or cost based, until very recently there were few norms for determining whether the costs or charges accumulated by the patient were in some sense too high or too low. Relative cost or relative efficiency had no effects on reimbursement rates.

Why does the reimbursement system look like this? For commercial insurers the answer probably depends on transactions costs. Any individual insurer covers a fairly small share of the individuals in any area and would find only a small share of the patients in any single hospital covered by one of its contracts.[19] Negotiating individual cost-based contracts with each hospital would be extremely costly relative to the number of patients the typical private carrier covers in that hospital in a year. Negotiating differential reimbursement rates among hospitals based on relative efficiency criteria would be even more costly. In this case, paying the posted charges may simply be the most economical thing to do. Furthermore, even if a private insurer felt that it could economically negotiate with individual hospitals, the individual insurer's small share of the total revenues of a hospital would tend to limit its bargaining power. The insurance carrier is likely to lose a lot more if a couple of hospitals stop taking assignment on its policies than the hospital is going to lose if those patients are forced to go elsewhere, especially if several hospitals come to a tacit understanding to restrict the ease of reimbursement from a particular carrier. In principle, private insurers could act collectively to negotiate better and more detailed reimbursement terms, but this kind of collective activity is almost certainly illegal under the antitrust laws.

Blue Cross, Medicare, and Medicaid are clearly in a much better position to negotiate cost-based contracts with individual hospitals and to impose other reimbursement restrictions to reduce inefficiencies. They are better able to exploit the economies of scale associated with cost-based reimbursement contracting, and hospitals are in a poor position to refuse to deal with them. The question is, why doesn't Blue Cross incorporate additional restrictions and monitoring arrangements into the reimbursement contracts that both reduce moral hazard problems and penalize inefficient providers? Two answers are possible. The negotiation and monitoring costs associated with more detailed reimbursement restrictions aimed at achieving these results may simply be too high. The transactions costs associated with reducing moral hazard and penalizing inefficiency while maintaining the risk-spreading benefits of insurance are simply higher than the efficiency gains that would ensue. Alternatively, it could be argued that Blue Cross plans have little incentive to behave this way because they are insulated from the threat that their competitors can do so efficiently and because such restrictions conflict with other objectives, including the welfare of hospitals and physicians. In short, Blue Cross plans may not be acting competitively and may not be pursuing all opportunities for providing the most efficient menu of insurance contracts that is economically feasible.[20]

Whether reimbursement is based on actual costs or accumulated charges is really not the fundamental issue in the effects of third-party reimbursement on the behavior and performance of consumers and providers in the hospital system. The critical characteristic of a general pass-through reimbursement scheme is that it provides few norms to constrain the types of available care or the costs of providing that care. It is almost as if the federal government offered to reimburse every citizen for 90 percent of his expenditures on clothing without any further critieria on the amount, types, or costs of clothing purchased. Consumers would have incentives to purchase a lot of clothing, they would have incentives to purchase very expensive clothing, and they would have no incentives to shop for the best deal. Similarly, suppliers would have little incentive to offer lower-cost clothing on to run their stores efficiently. There would be little incentive for price competition. The government would end up paying a very big bill, although the population would be very well clothed indeed.

The combination of extensive, nearly complete insurance coverage combined with a reimbursement system that essentially pays whatever resource expenditures are incurred by the hospitals leads to hospital behavior that is at least on the surface, a potential source of considerable inefficiency. Under prevailing institutional arrangements there is almost no price competition between hospitals serving a particular area, and no natural selection mechanism exists to constrain hospitals that produce inefficiently. Consider the insured patient. Even if there are large differences in the costs of care among hospitals, with a very low coinsurance rate the patient has little reason to base his choice on cost.[21] The patient with complete insurance coverage will almost certainly base his selection on factors other than the costs of supplying care. Indeed, to the extent that there are good substitution possibilities between outpatient and inpatient care, he is always going to choose inpatient care rather than outpatient care if the former is covered by insurance and the latter is not, even if outpatient care is less costly. Similarly, by basing reimbursement on individual hospital costs or charges without any independent normative criteria, the insurance firms do not provide independent incentives for hospitals to minimize costs. Thus the traditional contractual relationships between patient and insurer and between insurer and provider provide no independent cost-minimizing incentives.

The combination of complete insurance and full cost reimbursement to individual nonprofit hospitals restricts the normal market forces that stimulate cost-minimizing behavior, given current technology and input prices as well as process innovations that might reduce the costs of providing diagnostic and therapeutic techniques. But hospitals still compete with one another. All models of hospital objectives imply that hospitals prefer to have more rather than fewer patients and to provide a wider range of diagnostic and therapeutic services and higher-quality services.[22] If a hospital cannot attract patients (through their physicians) by reducing the cost of care (via price competition), then it will try to use other instruments. The most effective way to attract patients and physicians is to increase the scope and quality of services that are available.[23] In competing for patients, hospitals are likely to resort to quality competition as characterized by the availability of a full range of diagnostic and therapeutic services, more intensive care of patients, and amenities.

Thus if one hospital in an area has a CT scanner, other hospitals in the area are going to want to have CT scanners to attract patients and physicians, even if, because of economies of scale, it makes economic sense for only one hospital in any area to have this service. Neither patient-selection incentives with complete insurance nor traditional reimbursement formulas constrain this kind of behavior. The natural tendency is thus to increase the intensity of care and improve amenities. This behavior is intensified by independent objectives that nonprofit hospitals have to increase the scope and intensity of care or to pursue other objectives that often characterize nonprofit organizations not subject to the normal financial discipline of the market. Since physicians are the primary "gatekeepers" to the hospital, their preferences are also quite important and will be consistent with increasing the scope and quality of services, in both the interests of their patients and their own financial interests. This service rivalry and quality competition may be an important source of both static and dynamic inefficiency in the system. Any economic rents or supranormal profits that the hospital market might generate will be consumed by nonprice competition or in pursuit of individual hospital preferences for a larger range of services and more intensive care.

There is, therefore, another potential distortion associated with changes in the completeness of insurance contracts. Most analyses of the "optimal" insurance package assume that whatever is supplied is produced at minimum cost. However, as insurance contracts become more complete in the context of traditional reimbursement arrangements between insurers and hospitals, incentives for cost-minimizing behavior are reduced and incentives for service rivalry and other forms of nonprice competition increase.[24] These supply-side responses are likely to lead to the provision of hospital care at other than minimum cost. Furthermore, not only is hospital care likely to be provided inefficiently given prevailing technologies, but the insurance-reimbursement system is likely to encourage even more costly dynamic responses, in terms of a product innovation rate that is too high and a process innovation rate that is too low.

The Internal Organization of the Hospital

Our market imperfections perspective has subsumed the internal organization and internal behavior of the typical community hospital into a fairly simple objective function. Especially for evaluating the proposals for economic regulation, it is useful to develop a more complete picture of the internal organization of the hospital and how that organizational structure has evolved as a result of the hospital's traditional economic environment.

This view of the internal structure and organizational behavior of the hospital draws on work by Harris.[25] However, I try to provide a more detailed linkage between organizational structure and behavior and the economic environment in which hospitals operated during the late 1960s and early 1970s.[26] The hospital can be characterized by two primary but largely separate internal organizations: the hospital administration and the medical staff (including house staff and community physicians with admitting privileges). Physicians admit and treat patients essentially without the interference of the administrator. The administrator's role is to manage an organization whose basic function is to provide diagnostic, therapeutic, supervisory, and hotel-type resources for the physician's use. The medical staff is usually divided into medical specialties, while the administration supervises therapeutic and diagnostic services (laboratory, radiology departments) and support services (nursing care units, food, laundry). See figure 3.1. This organizational structure is also characterized by a particular command and control system: the physicians demand services that they feel are required for treating the patient, and the administrator endeavors to make the required resources available.

The role of insurance and prevailing third-party reimbursement policies is critical for understanding why this one-way command and control system has developed. Most hospital patients have

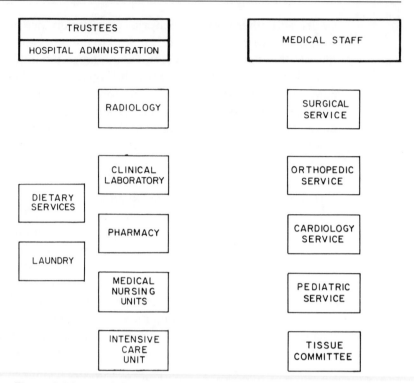

Figure 3.1 Internal Organization of a Hospital
Adapted from J.E. Harris. "The Internal Organization of Hospitals."
Bell Journal of Economics 8, no. 2 (Autumn 1977).

insurance with negligible coinsurance rates. For these patients the physician views resources as essentially free; the patient's budget provides little incentive to conserve resources. Similarly, the internal pricing and allocation system provides no independent incentives to the physician to take the cost of care into account; neither the physician nor his department faces an internal budgetary constraint. As a result, the physician demands services that are even marginally beneficial regardless of the associated resource costs. Indeed, from an agency perspective, the physician should demand all services that might be medically indicated without concern for broader economic consequences.

In principle, the hospital administrator could be confronted with a fairly inflexible budgetary constraint, which would make it impossible for him to satisfy all physician demands without incurring a deficit and throwing the hospital into bankruptcy. If this were the case, not all physicians' demands could be supplied, the administrator would have to reveal this supply-demand imbalance to physicians, and some institutional structure would have had to evolve to rationalize imbalances between supply and demand. However, the hospital reimbursement policies of the 1960s and early 1970s imposed only loose budgetary constraints, since third-party payers generally reimburse based on a cost-of-service formula or the posted charges for the individual hospital. Rather than allow a conflict between what the physicians demand and what the hospital can supply, the administrator endeavors to increase resource capabilities by building new facilities, hiring more staff, and adding new equipment under the assumption that the costs of additional supply will be reimbursed by third-party payers. Furthermore, with so large a proportion of the population covered by insurance policies that do not discriminate between high-cost and low-cost hospitals, any price competition that might otherwise put constraints on the administrator is eliminated. In short, a command and control system in which the physician demands and the hospital supplies does not encounter a fundamental conflict because the hospital is not subject to particularly stringent budgetary constraints. As long as the hospital can find the money to expand capacity by passing costs along to third-party payers, the potential conflict between hospital care "needs" and the costs of providing that care never arises.

Obviously, this description of the hospital is a simplified characterization of a much more complicated system. Some patients do not have extensive insurance coverage, budget constraints are not infinitely flexible, and mismatches between demand and supply sometimes do develop and must be resolved. However, I believe that this characterization represents a useful model of organizational structure and behavior over the period 1966–1975 prior to the imposition of regulatory and other financial constraints.

This conceptual framework provides a useful vehicle for viewing the static and dynamic elements of what is perceived to be a serious problem of resource misallocation and excessive costs in the hospital sector. A number of observations can be made.

1. This organizational structure, the associated command and control system, and the reimbursement system that sustains it lead to an organization with either weak administrators or administrators who consider it their job to build a bigger, more

sophisticated, and more prestigious hospital. The administrator interested primarily in organizational changes designed to reduce costs is not likely to survive long in this system. The physicians in the hospital dictate what the hospital will provide, and the administrator endeavors to ensure that there are resources to provide these services. Without the discipline of binding budgetary constraints or price competition among hospitals, the administrator has little incentive or leverage to affect the allocation of resources. Without a strong administrator with incentives to enforce cost-minimizing production decisions, organizational slack or x-inefficiency is likely to characterize the hospital. It is also unlikely that the hospital would attract the types of administrators who have the best capabilities to play an active role in promoting the efficient allocation of resources in the hospital, because the administrator traditionally has had little leverage to exert such authority.

2. Any sudden expansion of insurance coverage along with full cost reimbursement will lead to an increase in the demand for existing services. This increase in demand will be accommodated by increased expenditures by hospitals to meet that demand. Basic conflicts between demand and supply are likely to emerge only in the short run before capacity can be expanded to meet the new higher level of demand. Thus, without technological change, we would expect a sudden increase in insurance coverage and an associated shift in demand to lead to an associated increase in expenditures, with some lag, but not to a continuous increase in expenditures. Short-run supply constraints are likely to be dealt with by rough queuing of admissions because no mechanisms exist for more refined rationing.[27]

3. The tendency of hospitals to show long-term increases in real expenditures long after major changes in insurance coverage is a result of the dynamics of technical change in this sector. The introduction of new diagnostic and therapeutic techniques has been a fact in American hospitals for at least 30 years. How much of the expansion of the opportunity set is exogenous and how much is endogenous is difficult to determine. What is clear is that as the opportunity set expands, new diagnostic and therapeutic techniques are rapidly incorporated into the demands made by physicians. As long as there are minimal financial or regulatory constraints, the administrator can do little but provide the services

that the physicians want. His only argument for not doing so is the "social good" rather than the welfare of the actual patients treated in the hospital.

4. Even if we could convince the hospital administrator that this entire process had unattractive social cost-benefit characteristics and the administrator could exert enough leverage within the hospital to deny requests for more services, external contraints also inhibit such behavior. In most areas of the country several hospitals serve overlapping patient populations. If physicians cannot get what they want from one hospital, they will try to get it from another. A single administrator oriented toward cost control and wider considerations of social efficiency may find his efforts rewarded with the departure of top physicians and their patients. This effect is unlikely to gain for the administrator the admiration of the hospital's trustees. For the hospital to survive and grow, the administrator must endeavor to meet or beat the competition. He cannot do it by providing care at lower cost so he must do it by providing the services that can attract physicians and their patients.

This organizational structure and behavior of hospitals is not a consequence of the hospital's being different in some fundamental sense from other complex organizations. An organizational structure for allocating resources without regard to costs and values has evolved because the economic environment in which hospitals function does not penalize this type of behavior. Indeed, to the extent that there is a natural selection process in this system, it reinforces organizational structure and behavior that ignore costs and vigorously pursue more and better hospital services. We get a system where the physician is king and the administrator is either weak or is a builder himself. Any conflicts for society between the value and costs of services are not reflected in the way that the internal organization of the hospital has evolved to manage supply and demand decisions.

Any efforts to alter the behavior and performance of the hospital sector as a whole—whether improved market incentives or administrative regulation—must imply fundamental changes in the internal organization of the hospital. The problems of institutional change may be most acute in a system that relies on supply-side constraints imposed by regulatory authorities that do not affect the individual incentives of patients and physicians directly.

The Role of the Physician

The physician is the primary intermediary between the patient and the hospital and is largely responsible for the kinds of services a patient receives once he is admitted to the hospital. The physician is normally thought of as the patient's agent in this system. Ideally, the physician possesses the training and knowledge to apply medical technology in the best interest of the patient. Clearly, the kind of insurance and reimbursement system that we have in the United States conforms nicely with the objectives that the ideal physician is taught to have: Do whatever is possible to resolve your patient's medical problem without regard to cost or even cost effectiveness. If patients had only very incomplete insurance, physicians would continually find themselves confronted with the difficult problem of trading off beneficial health care against the patient's ability and willingness to pay for it. The prevalence of low deductible insurance among a very large segment of the population relieves the physician of making such choices. The insured patient faces little financial constraint, the hospital faces little financial constraint, and the well-trained and knowledgeable physician can practice his profession to the best of his ability without financial constraints. One could, of course, conceptualize a physician who provided care only up to the point where expected benefits and costs are equal on the margin. But the physician is not trained to do this and faces no incentives to do this under traditional institutional arrangements. Nor would his insured patient want him to do this unless insurance institutions enabled him to obtain insurance at a lower price commensurate with the reduction in moral hazard associated with choosing a more restrictive physician.[28] We therefore should not expect the physician to act independently to reduce the inherent inefficiencies in the system. To the extent that he acts on his perceptions of the best interest of the individually insured patients, he provides the knowledge that ensures the realization of these inefficiencies.

Medical science is not at a point where there are always clear and well-defined linkages between particular diagnostic and therapeutic courses of action and health care outcomes. In one dimension physicians may face a clear ordering of diagnostic and therapeutic alternatives regarding their expected value to the patient. In another dimension, as a result of conflicting scientific evidence and uncertain outcomes, alternative courses of action may be almost indistinguishable with regard to expected benefits. On the first dimension the failure of costs to play a role in the physician's decision making leads to the provision of the "best" care. In the second, the lack of cost considerations provide few incentives for physicians to engage in cost-effectiveness analysis (rather than a more difficult cost-benefit analysis), which would tend to push diagnostic and therapeutic decisions toward the least costly of the high-quality alternatives.

Given prevailing insurance institutions, we should not expect the physician to act to reduce moral hazard problems, since his patient's insurance contract implicitly assumes that he will not. Teaching the physician the principles of cost-benefit analysis will not help much. The physician who provided less care on the grounds that the expected benefits of additional care, while positive, were less than the costs to society of providing such care, would soon lose all his patients unless there were some mechanism to return any associated resource savings to the patient in the form of lower premiums. Thus we can certainly conceptualize an individual consumer's choosing an insurance contract with a negligible coinsurance rate but with the restriction that care be provided only by physicians and hospitals who do so only if it satisfies some reasonable cost-benefit criterion. The patient's incentive to choose this type of contract would be a lower premium. The incentives of insurance companies to provide such contracts is limited, however, by their ability to ensure that medical decisions of physicians mitigate moral hazard.

A health maintenance organization (HMO) has some of these characteristics. An individual who enrolls in an HMO generally has an insurance package that is at least as complete as that provided under a typical private insurance plan, if we view completeness in terms of what the patient must pay out of pocket. Because HMOs face fixed annual budget constraints, however, and must engage in price competition with private insurance plans to attract enrollees, they have strong incentives to constrain the supply of hospital care. They may constrain supply through internal organizational allocational mechanisms based on incentives, specific criteria, or even queues. The HMO package may actually increase the demand for care by patients, but the HMO organization has incentives to ration the care that is actually available. A patient with a particular medical problem may be hospitalized if he has a conventional insurance contract, but an identical patient may be treated on a less costly (and perhaps but not necessarily lower quality) outpatient basis if he is enrolled in an HMO. To the extent that HMOs are successful in rationing care with unattractive cost-benefit ratios, they may be quite successful in reducing moral hazard problems and can simultaneously offer patients lower coinsurance rates and lower premiums. Of course, in reality, the HMO contract may be in a sense less complete than the conventional insurance package because it involves more screening and rationing of ex post consumption decisions, which go beyond simple cost effectiveness.

The spread of health maintenance organizations and the development of similar organizational or contractual arrangements has been limited. The reasons include the tax subsidies associated with employer-provided insurance plans; the ways in which employees pay for their group plans; differences in consumer preferences regarding health care delivery alternatives; potentially unattractive characteristics of health maintenance organizations for some individuals; transactions and monitoring costs incurred in constraining patient, physician, and hospital behavior; and perhaps monopolistic restrictions that make the formation of such alternatives unnecessarily difficult. In addition, physicians may find the traditional fee-for-service system more congenial because it allows them to practice without significant financial or administrative restrictions on the care they can provide or because the prevailing system generates higher physician incomes. The increased efficiency that HMOs may be able to achieve results from their ability to constrain the availability of certain types of care to certain types of patients. This supply constraint implies an inherent "excess demand," which individuals may be willing to accept if the premiums are low enough or if the increased availability of other types of care more than compensates for the potential restrictions.

To summarize, we should not expect physicians, aside from those practicing in HMOs or similar organizations, to behave independently to reduce moral hazard problems. Indeed, under traditional insurance and reimbursement institutions, the physician is in the position to increase the inefficiencies that may characterize this system. Physicians may have personal financial incentives to prescribe more care than is beneficial to the patient. That the insured patient pays little or nothing on the margin may encourage such behavior. To the extent that this agency problem is important, more resources will be expended without producing any additional patient benefits and perhaps causing harm. Malpractice laws and internal hospital review committees may help deter the most serious distortions that actually harm the patient; but along that portion of the benefit curve where marginal benefits are very small, we can expect that the physician's financial interests will lead him to extend the quantity and quality of care as far as possible.

The Insurance Industry

Additional distortions may arise as a result of imperfect competition among health insurers or monopolistic restrictions on entry and pricing of innovative hospital insurance plans and health care delivery schemes. Most theoretical and empirical analyses of the provision of insurance assume that hospital insurance packages are generated by a competitive market process. This assumption is a candidate for careful scrutiny.

Private hospital insurance is provided by nonprofit Blue Cross plans and by private commercial insurance companies, usually life insurance companies. Approximately half of the insurance benefits are provided by Blue Cross plans and half by commercial insurers, although this proportion varies considerably from state to state (table 3.1).[29] Since Blue Cross coverage is normally provided by a single Blue Cross organization in any area and since commercial insurance is provided by many different insurance firms, Blue

Table 3.1 Private Hospital Insurance in the United States, 1977

Type of Plan	Gross Enrollment[a] (thousands)	Benefits Paid ($ billions)	Operating Expenses/ Premiums[b] (percent)
Blue Cross, Blue Shield	85,101	11.5	6.8
Commercial Insurers	117,906	11.2	18.6
Independent Plans	15,600	1.8	7.0

[a] Includes persons enrolled in more than one plan. Net coverage is about 85 percent of gross enrollment.
[b] Based on experience for all medical insurance, not just hospital insurance.
Source: M. S. Carroll and R. H. Arnett III. "Private Health Insurance Plans in 1977; Coverage, Enrollment, and Financial Experience." *Health Care Financing Review*, 1, no. 2 (Fall 1979), pp. 3–22.

Cross always has a much larger market share than the next largest private insurance carrier. Typically Blue Cross has a share of 50 percent, and the largest commercial insurer has a share of perhaps 10 percent. In most cases the local Blue Cross organization is the dominant insurance carrier.

Blue Cross plans were initially created during the depression largely under the auspices of groups of hospitals or hospital associations in particular areas of the country.[30] Although many motivations for the development of hospital service benefit plans have been suggested, the hospitals' interests in developing a market for their services and in getting paid for the cost of providing these services was certainly very important. Blue Cross plans were traditionally sanctioned and approved by the American Hospital Association (AHA). Until 1972 the Blue Cross name and the Blue Cross emblem were the property of the AHA.[31] The extensive control that hospitals had over Blue Cross plans during their formative years has apparently eroded considerably. Most Blue Cross plans now have boards of directors composed predominantly of public members who are neither affiliated with hospitals nor members of the health care profession. The real source of control over Blue Cross plans and alleged tendencies to pursue the interests of providers rather than consumers remains a subject of lively, and unresolved, debate.[32] There is considerable evidence of growing friction between some Blue Cross plans and the hospitals in their area as the plans have begun to initiate cost containment efforts. The entire system has been changing, and the very strong control that hospitals had over the Blue Cross plans 20 or 30 years ago has eroded as the composition of boards of directors has changed and competition from commercial insurers has increased. Nevertheless, some analysts believe that participating hospitals still have substantial control,[33] and this control is thought to affect Blue Cross objectives and behavior.

Blue Cross plans are private nonprofit organizations that normally operate under special state-enabling legislation. Along with their nonprofit status, this legislation grants the plans special tax savings and in some cases special regulatory treatment unavailable to commercial insurers. In several states, especially the older industrialized states, Blue Cross plans reimburse hospitals under cost-based reimbursement contracts. In effect these contracts allow them to pay for services at lower rates than patients insured by commercial insurance plans must pay. Obviously, other things equal, if Blue Cross pays lower rates than its competitors, it is likely to have a significant advantage in competing for group and individual coverage. In fact, Blue Cross market shares tend to be higher in states that have such reimbursement arrangements. To the extent that Blue Cross has power, through its cost advantages, its linkages with hospitals, or its size, to define the basic form for hospital insurance contracts, it could affect the kinds of insurance contracts available to consumers in the market as well as the contractual relationships between insurers and providers. Given its size, Blue Cross should be in an excellent position to exploit all available instruments to reduce moral hazard problems through its contractual relationships with consumers, their surrogate groups, and health care providers. The question is whether Blue Cross is exploiting these opportunities to the fullest or is pursuing other objectives with limited constraints from competing insurance firms.

Although these issues have not been investigated extensively in the literature, we can point to some evidence on each side of this question. Frech and Ginsburg (1978) have argued that the Blue Cross uses its cost advantages to promote more extensive insurance coverage, that some of the cost advantage is consumed as organizational slack, and that hospital costs are higher in states with Blue Cross plans that have very large market shares than in states where Blue Cross has a small market share. On the other hand, Blue Cross plans have lower loadings on their policies, appear to be able to process claims more cheaply than the commercial insurers can, and in some states have instituted innovative cost containment schemes. However, it remains unclear whether Blue Cross has moved as quickly or gone as far as it could to use its size and cost advantages to provide more efficient insurance policies and reimbursement contracts.

With all the advantages of the Blue Cross plans, one wonders how the commercial insurers are able to compete. The opportunity for competition, and what appears to be active price competition between commercial insurers and Blue Cross and among commercial insurers, are attributable to a number of characteristics of Blue Cross premium and contracting policies. First, as Frech and Ginsburg have noted, and as Blue Cross acknowledges, Blue Cross plans tend to offer relatively complete service benefit contracts with small deductibles and copayment provisions. They offer extensive inpatient service coverage and tend to avoid offering less

complete inpatient insurance packages. Blue Cross argues that
people should have this kind of insurance, and it is their philos-
ophy to provide relatively complete inpatient insurance.[34] (This
type of coverage may also be less costly to process.) Commercial
insurers can thus compete by offering different levels of coverage
and different types of coverage, including different mixes of inpatient and outpatient coverage. Second, Blue Cross plans have
traditionally based premiums on community risk characteristics
rather than the risk experience of particular groups. This has meant
that all groups in any area paid the same insurance rates regardless
of the individual risks of the groups. This policy has provided an
opportunity for commercial insurers to provide lower-cost coverage to groups that had better risk characteristics than the community as a whole. More recently, in response to this competition,
Blue Cross plans in some states have begun to use experience
rating or merely to administer reimbursement for large self-insured
business firms. Finally, commercial insurers sell group life insurance policies, run retirement plans, and in some cases compete
for groups by offering an attractive package of insurance services
for a company's employees. Recently, some Blue Cross plans have
gotten into the life insurance business to compete on the same
basis with the commercial insurers.

Our understanding of the nature and extent of competition in
the hospital insurance market remains incomplete. In many states
price competition among insurers appears to be fairly active especially for group plans. However, there remains some question
about the ability of Blue Cross to pursue goals that are not unduly
influenced by providers. Too much provider influence may result
in restricted policy options and the erosion of cost advantages by
organizational slack. The presence of an aggressive commercial
insurance industry, however, certainly puts substantial constraints
on Blue Cross's independent abilities to behave monopolistically.

Of more antitrust concern are provider actions aimed at restricting innovative insurance and reimbursement arrangements
and the creation of more efficient organizational forms for delivering hospital care. Over the years there have been allegations
that the formation of group practices and HMOs has sometimes
been restricted by state medical societies.[35] Goldberg and Greenberg (1978) provide a fascinating historical example of the evolution of competing cost-concious, prepaid hospital association
insurance plans in Oregon in the 1930s. Organized medicine in

Oregon fought these insurance plans. First it expelled participating physicians from medical associations. Then it sponsored an alternative state-wide insurance system in which physicians could participate and which enabled them to refuse to deal with hospital-sponsored insurance plans that constrained reimbursement rates and services. This led to the eventual demise of the hospital-sponsored loans oriented toward cost control.

Aside from a few interesting case studies such as this one, there has been relatively little systematic analysis of the prevalence of similar types of anticompetitive behavior. Such a comprehensive study would certainly be worthwhile. All we can say now is that such anticompetitive behavior is possible and could severely restrict the efficient provision of both hospital insurance and hospital care.

In summary, the efficiency of the insurance policies supplied by the market requires that competition among insurance firms yield a menu of health insurance options that reflects the preferences of consumers and that all economical opportunities to mitigate moral hazard problems are exploited. This result is more likely in a competitive insurance market, with price competition and free entry, than in a market in which monopolistic restrictions inhibit price competition, entry, and innovation. The health insurance industry has become more competitive over time, but lingering restrictions on full and fair competition may remain, and every effort should be made to eliminate them.

Quantifying the Inefficiencies

This set of structural and behavioral characteristics has led many economists to conclude that the hospital sector is characterized by excessive demands for services and a variety of distortions on the supply side. The major source of distortion on both the supply and demand sides is an insurance and reimbursement system that has virtually eliminated all fiscal constraints on insured patients and hospital care providers. The major agents in the system—patient, physician, and hospital—have little incentive to take the cost of care into account when making consumption and production decisions. Price competition between hospitals is all but eliminated and is supplemented by vigorous quality competition much like that experienced in price-constrained airline markets.[36] We tend to get an overutilization of hospital services, duplication of hospital facilities engendered by nonprice competition and leading to a failure to fully exploit economies of scale, an excessive rate of technological change biased toward product rather than process innovations, and organizational slack.

Quantifying these distortions in terms of efficiency losses and excessive expenditures is not an easy task. Inquiry into the types and magnitudes of distortions requires some norm for comparison—inefficient compared with what? It is easy to conceptualize an ideal system where information and transactions costs are zero. All moral hazard problems as well as incremental demand and supply distortions then become candidate inefficiencies. But this basis for comparison is not particularly useful, except perhaps to structure a more sophisticated inquiry. Information costs and transactions costs are not zero, "perfect" insurance contracts cannot be written, and what appear to be inefficiencies compared with some abstract ideal may in fact represent the best that we can do given the economic factors that characterize transactions in the real world. For any particular potential source of inefficiency, we must continually ask whether proposed policy initiatives can actually improve welfare—considering costs, hospital care demand and supply distortions, and the risk-spreading benefits and risk-bearing costs associated with changes in the system.

What we can do is identify precisely where we might expect inefficiencies. Then we can evaluate alternative regulatory mechanisms in terms of the potential size of the distortions and the likelihood that any policy instrument can reduce their costs without imposing other offsetting costs.

At least five potentially undesirable performance characteristics of the hospital sector are worth focusing on in considering proposed regulatory mechanisms:

1. Excessive demand and consumption of diagnostic and therapeutic techniques given a fixed opportunity set of such techniques.
2. Excessive rates of introduction and diffusion of new diagnostic and therapeutic techniques.
3. Duplication of hospital facilities (both general hospital beds and specific diagnostic and treatment facilities) resulting in a failure to exploit fully all economies of scale given the prevailing demand for services.
4. Organizational slack, or x-inefficiency.
5. Too low a rate of cost-reducing process innovations.

These five performance categories represent two types of inefficiency: a failure to provide the services demanded at minimum cost and too much in the way of hospital services being demanded and supplied, even if provided at minimum cost. In a sense these potential performance failures are the symptoms of the problem rather than its causes. In the evaluation of alternative regulatory policies, it is often useful to examine both the symptoms and the causes.

The rapid growth rate in hospital expenditures and the increasing burden of this growth on government payment programs has been a primary "political" motivation for regulation. How much of the increase in hospital expenditures can be associated with one or more of the types of inefficiency mentioned before? We do not know with any precision. Merely comparing changes in expenditures with changes in aggregate economic activity or changes in the cost per patient-day with the consumer price index is not particularly meaningful. Over this period the population and per capita income have grown, demographic characteristics have changed, insurance coverage has increased enormously, real wages for hospital employees have increased, and, most important, the "product" that hospitals deliver has undergone profound changes. Comparing the current price of a day in the hospital with the price 20 years ago is like comparing the price of a 1980 Ford with the price of a model T. Thinking about the issues of resource misallocation merely in the context of price inflation is completely misleading. To identify the types and magnitudes of these inefficiencies and to separate increases in expenditures that are in some sense optimal from expenditures that represent waste and inefficiency requires a much deeper inquiry.

The only work in the literature that yields fairly comprehensive quantitative results is that of Feldstein.[37] His work has focused on the effects of increasing insurance coverage on hospital expenditures and has tried to evaluate the effects that tax subsidies to health insurance and associated reductions in the average coinsurance rate have had on hospital expenditures and consumer welfare. Feldstein finds that a very large fraction of the increase in hospital expenditures can be explained by reductions in the aggregate coinsurance rate and that tax incentives have kept the aggregate coinsurance rate below the optimal level. Thus comparing the actual coinsurance rate with the "optimal" coinsurance rate yields values for the welfare losses and increased expenditures associated with excessive insurance coverage.[38] The analysis leads to estimated optimal coinsurance rates that are substantially larger than prevailing coinsurance rates.[39] Feldstein's estimates of the welfare losses and increased expenditures on hospital care due to excessive insurance coverage amount to several billion dollars per year. This work is subject to a number of theoretical and empirical criticisms, some of which have been discussed by Harris (1979b), and the numerical results must be considered to be characterized by considerable uncertainty.[40] The results depend on particular assumptions about consumer preferences as well as uncertain empirical relationships between the average coinsurance rate and the demand and supply of hospital services. However legitimate the criticisms, Feldstein's work represents the only comprehensive empirical effort to assess the costs of increased insurance and the welfare losses induced by tax distortions.

More frequently those who argue that there are large inefficiencies in the hospital system use other types of evidence. For example, wide cross-sectional disparities in surgical rates, hospital beds per capita, average length of hospital stay, physicians per capita, and cost per admission (tables 3.2, 3.3) without any sig-

Table 3.2 Selected State Data on Supply and Utilization (per thousand population)

	Beds	Physicians	ALS (days)	Admissions	Surgical Operations	Percentage 65+
Alabama	4.8	109	7.1	186	77.4	10.8
California	3.8	222	6.6	141	71.6	10.0
Connecticut	3.5	229	7.5	134	75.7	10.9
Florida	5.0	192	7.5	174	81.0	17.1
Georgia	4.3	130	6.4	169	78.4	9.0
Illinois	4.9	170	8.0	171	80.1	10.6
Iowa	4.3	116	7.5	189	82.8	13.0
Louisiana	4.5	138	6.4	181	83.6	9.3
Massachusetts	4.5	245	8.5	152	86.5	11.9
Montana	4.6	122	6.4	173	75.5	10.4
New York	4.4	258	9.8	147	74.5	11.6
Oregon	3.7	178	6.2	148	84.2	11.5
Texas	4.6	140	6.6	171	78.0	9.6
Utah	3.0	161	5.2	148	74.4	7.7

Source: *Selected Community Hospital Indicators 1977*. Chicago: American Hospital Association, 1979.

Table 3.3 Regional Variations in Surgical Rates (surgical operations per hundred thousand population)

Type of Surgery	Northeast	North Central	South	West
Neurosurgery	150.6	215.9	162.6	223.1
Tonsillectomy	178.8	322.7	245.7	271.9
Prostatectomy	146.2	176.6	107.7	129.6
Hysterectomy	205.7	317.5	371.1	270.8
Varicose veins	39.7	32.7	19.4	23.1

Source: *Utilization of Short Stay Hospitals, 1978*. National Center for Health Statistics, Series 13, Number 46, DHEW Publication No. PHS 80-1797. Washington, D.C.: U.S. Government Printing Office, 1980.

nificant associated differences in health status are often pointed to as evidence that additional resource expenditures on hospital care yield at best marginal health benefits.[41] Difficulty in measuring health status and differences in the demographic and health characteristics of the population necessarily raise problems in drawing strong implications from such observations. The general thrust of these observations, however, is consistent with Feldstein's studies and with the observation that as insurance coverage becomes more complete, we should observe an increasing disparity between benefits and costs on the margin. Unfortunately, without making some judgment about the appropriate trade-off between the risk-spreading benefits of insurance, the efficiency losses associated with moral hazard, and the efficiency with which current institutions constrain the behavior that leads to a moral hazard problem, it is difficult to make welfare judgments from such observations. To use these observations as a motivation for policies to promote institutional change one must either believe, as Feldstein does, that the system generates excessive insurance coverage or that alternative institutional arrangements can constrain demand and supply behavior to reduce inefficiencies without incurring offsetting increases in risk-bearing costs.

These general observations of regional and even international diversity can be supplemented by specific studies of the utilization of particular diagnostic or treatment techniques. Several retrospective studies of surgical procedures indicate that a significant fraction of patients are operated on without appropriate indications.[42] The figures obtained for particular procedures vary widely, however, and the entire approach has been characterized by enormous controversy.[43] Similarly, some have tried to interpret high nonconfirmation rates in surgical second opinion programs as an indication that a significant fraction of the surgery performed in the United States is unnecessary.[44] But these results may be also subject to serious misinterpretation.[45]

Similar studies of diagnostic procedures have also been made. Studies of the routine use of chest X rays and of laboratory tests indicate that for some classes of patients they produce no useful diagnostic information.[46] Studies of CT scanning have yielded conflicting results regarding both benefits and costs. Despite the controversy, the weight of the evidence seems to be that CT scanning is beneficial for many patients and may actually save money for some classes of patients.[47] These studies show that on the margin diagnostic and therapeutic techniques are used to a point where the expected benefits are very small or even zero. Once again, the question is whether there are ways to control a moral hazard problem, or a moral hazard problem compounded by excessive insurance, without changing the coinsurance rate. In the first case we must investigate whether there are better ways to control patient or provider behavior so that ex post consumption and production decisions are more efficient without sacrificing the risk-spreading benefits of insurance. To the extent that excessive insurance coverage reinforces this problem, we must be willing either to consider changing the incentives to purchase too much insurance or to devise mechanisms that can improve welfare accounting for both the ex ante and ex post efficiency considerations.

Finally, a few studies have looked at the supply side of the system in an effort to determine whether current patterns of care can be provided more efficiently. McClure has examined the cost of excess beds.[48] Finkler has examined the savings that might be achieved by eliminating duplication in open-heart surgery and cardiac catheterization facilities.[49] Schwartz and Joskow examined the theoretical savings that might be achieved through facility consolidation indicated by the federal guidelines for CT scanners, open-heart surgery facilities, therapeutic radiology facilities, and general hospital beds.[50] They found that even the theoretical savings were surprisingly small and that the net savings are negligible after accounting for administrative costs and the additional travel costs of patients. Unlike the other evidence, however, the evidence on facility duplication and other inefficiencies in supply in principle require (at least at the extremes) much less difficult welfare judgments. If current patterns of care are provided at other than minimum cost, any changes that can economically reduce the costs of providing this care are pure welfare gains and do not involve a sacrifice of either ex ante or ex post benefits, real or perceived. Even here we run into practical complications if the elimination of duplicated facilities requires patients to travel longer distances for care. Travel costs must be considered as well as reductions in the quality of care to trauma patients who must travel farther and have treatment delayed longer than would otherwise be the case. Both may be difficult to estimate precisely.

While the available quantitative evidence on inefficiencies in the hospital sector does not allow us to make precise estimates of the five types of inefficiencies mentioned earlier, individually or in the aggregate, it does lead to some useful conclusions. First, there are significant inefficiencies in the system that amount to billions of dollars in expenditures per year. Second, the bulk of these inefficiencies are associated with excessive demand and consumption of diagnostic and therapeutic services and excessive rates of diffusion and utilization of new diagnostic and therapeutic techniques. Third, inefficiencies associated with facility duplication and organizational slack are real but are quantitatively less significant than the inefficiencies associated with excessive consumption.

Occupancy Rates and Excess Capacity

The rhetoric that accompanied recent federal efforts to institute a pervasive regulatory scheme to contain hospital costs painted a very different picture of the relative magnitudes of the different types of inefficiencies in the hospital system. In particular, there was considerable reliance on very large estimates of waste and inefficiency associated with facility duplication and various forms of organizational slack. For example Secretary of Health, Education, and Welfare Joseph Califano testified that at least $7 billion per year in expenditures were attributable to only a few of the sources of this type of waste.[51] Of particular importance were savings attributed to the elimination of general excess capacity in the hospital sector.

Much of the discussion of facility duplication and general excess capacity in the hospital sector relies on observations about the average annual occupancy rate of hospitals. The average annual occupancy rate is given by the number of actual inpatient days (admissions times average length of stay) divided by the number of available inpatient days (the number of hospital beds times 365 days). For example, for a 200-bed hospital with an average length of stay of 7.5 days and 7,300 admissions per year, the number of actual inpatient days is 54,750 (7,300 times 7.5) and the number of available inpatient days is 73,000 (200 times 365). This hospital has an average occupancy rate of 75 percent (54,750 divided by 73,000). Actual average annual occupancy rates at the state level vary from about 65 percent to over 80 percent, and the variation at the individual hospital level is even wider.

It has become routine among hospital planners and those who claim that there is much excess capacity to argue that average occupancy rates below some ideal value (usually somewhere between 80 percent and 90 percent) indicate the presence of excess capacity.[52] It is my view that raw data on average annual occupancy rates are not, in and of themselves, meaningful measures of excess capacity and that such figures should not be relied on to draw any general conclusions about excess capacity. These ideal occupancy rates are both arbitrary and meaningless.[53]

The actual occupancy rate achieved by a hospital with a given number of beds depends on a number of characteristics of the utilization of hospital services. The most important are the day-to-day fluctuations of admissions and discharges within a week, seasonal fluctuations of admissions throughout the year, the average length of stay of the patients admitted to the hospital, and the utilization of independent distinctive patient facilities (general medical surgical, intensive care, pediatric, maternity) that make up the hospital.

Day-to-Day Variations.
Hospitals normally have the largest proportion of their beds full during the week, especially during the first four days of the week. Occupancy rates fall toward the end of the week and stay low on weekends (figure 3.2).

Seasonal Variations.
Hospital admissions reflect seasonal differences in the incidence of illnesses requiring hospitalization and vacation periods. Admissions are highest during the winter months, lower in the summer, and very low around Christmas (figure 3.3).[54]

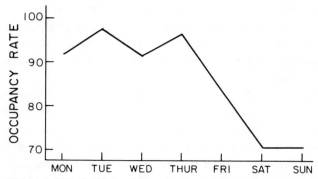

Figure 3.2 Daily Fluctuations in Occupancy, Peak Week for a Typical
Community Hospital
Adapted from Joskow (1980)

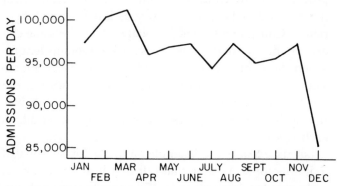

Figure 3.3 Monthly Fluctuations in Hospital Admissions
Adapted from Joskow (1980)

Average Length of Stay.

Length of stay varies with the type of patient and with the region
for patients with similar characteristics. The regional differences
have persisted for a long time and appear to reflect differences
in medical practice among the states. The average length of stay
is longer in the East than in the West.

Admissions Patterns.

Most hospitals and physicians attempt to concentrate elective admissions at the beginning of the week. Early-week admissions
combined with a median patient stay of less than five days and

the concentration of diagnostic and therapeutic services early in a patient's stay allow hospitals to operate with substantially reduced staffing on weekends. This policy accommodates typical five-day work weeks and minimizes overtime payments for hospital staff.

Let's consider a simple example to see the difficulties that arise from trying to draw inferences about excess capacity from average occupancy rate data. Assume that we have a 200-bed hospital that treats only elective patients with a length of stay of exactly five days. Assume further that patients are always admitted on Sunday evening and discharged on Friday morning and that the hospital admits exactly 200 patients each week. This hospital would have all beds full five days per week and would be empty on the weekends. It would have an average occupancy rate of about 70 percent. To admit additional patients, however, the hospital would have to add bed capacity as long as it maintained this admissions policy. Consider a second hospital with all the same characteristics except that it treats patients with an average length of stay of seven days, but admits only 190 patients each Sunday evening. This hospital would have an average occupancy rate of 95 percent. Yet this hospital has excess capacity even though it's occupancy rate is higher, since it can accommodate 10 additional patients each week.

Let us expand the example to allow for seasonal fluctuations in admissions. Assume that our first hospital admits 200 patients per week for 26 weeks and 175 patients per week for 26 weeks. This hospital now has a 67 percent occupancy rate. Yet this hospital can accommodate no additional patients during the peak period of the year without adding capacity. Although it can accommodate additional patients during the off-peak periods, a merger with another hospital would not change total bed capacity requirements unless the second hospital had different peaking characteristics.

Finally, assume that our first sample hospital is composed of a 150-bed medical-surgical unit and 50-bed obstetrical unit. Assume that the medical-surgical unit treats patients with five-day stays and admits them on Sundays uniformly throughout the year. Assume that the obstetrical unit admits 50 patients for 12 weeks and 30 patients for 40 weeks, reflecting seasonal variations in births. The medical-surgical unit has a 70 percent occupancy rate and the obstetrical unit has a 50 percent occupancy rate. The hospital as a whole has an occupancy rate of only 65 percent. Yet there is no opportunity to accommodate additional medical-surgical patients at any time and no excess capacity during peak periods for the obstetrical unit.

These examples demonstrate that no general conclusions can be drawn regarding the relationship between average occupancy rates and excess capacity. Our first hospital could reduce bed capacity while treating the same number of patients per year only by trying to shift admissions from peak periods to off-peak periods. The hospital might try an admissions policy that allows weekend utilization and admissions on any day of the week. (Both are required since there are only two weekend days but a five-day length of stay.) This shift could not be accomplished without cost, however. Although the shift would reduce required bed capacity, the hospital would have to increase weekend staffing, require physicians to be ready to admit patients seven days a week, inconvenience patients, and complicate admissions scheduling. Whether the savings outweigh the costs is unclear, and the notion of excess capacity becomes much more complicated. Where we have seasonal variations in admissions we can queue patients to reduce peak capacity requirements. This obviously changes the quality of care available to patients, since there is normally some value to prompt treatment. Again, whether the costs of such a strategy outweigh the benefits is unclear, and the notion of excess capacity becomes complex because we are effectively changing the quality of the product the hospital is offering.

Given fluctuating patient loads, length of stay, admissions policies, and distinctive patient facilities, a proper analysis of excess capacity is complex. The problem of determining the ideal number of beds and the ideal occupancy rate becomes even more complicated because of the randomness in admission and length of stay. Aside from general daily and seasonal fluctuations as well as differences in length of stay and organizational characteristics, there is also considerable uncertainty about how many patients will seek admission at any one time and how long any particular patient will stay. Faced with stochastic demands, a hospital must decide how much reserve capacity to have and with what probability it wants to turn patients away if the hospital is full. These random factors are of special concern for emergency admissions and for admissions that cannot be deferred for very long, such as obstetrical admissions. A hospital's decision about capacity depends on the mean and variance of the random demand and the cost of turning patients away. Whether hospitals have too much or too little capacity depends on a complete evaluation of the costs and benefits of different probabilities of turning patients away, the value of applying different queuing disciplines, and adaptations in admissions procedures. As long as patient arrivals are roughly random, however, and other things equal, a larger hospital should be better able than a smaller hospital to achieve a specific turnaway probability with a higher occupancy rate (lower reserve margin), since the coefficient of variation of demand increases less than proportionally with the size of the hospital. Assuming that we can agree on an appropriate accommodation of uncertain patient demands by defining an optimal turnaway probability, equal turnaway probabilities therefore imply occupancy rates that vary with the size of the patient load on individual hospitals.

Naive efforts to identify excess capacity by examining average occupancy rates are unlikely to be fruitful, and estimates of easy savings based on incorrect use of average occupancy rate data must be discounted. Nearly 70 percent of the variation in occupancy rates by state can be explained by two variables: average length of stay and average number of beds per hospital. Equation 3.1 is a simple linear regression of state hospital occupancy rates against a constant, the average length of stay, and the average size of hospitals in each state for 1978.

$$\text{Occupancy rate} = 0.49 + 0.02(\text{average length of stay})$$
$$(12.7) \quad (3.1)$$
$$+ 0.006(\text{beds per hospital}), \tag{3.1}$$
$$(6.4)$$

$$(t\text{ - statistics in parentheses})$$
$$R^2 = 0.69.$$

The empirical relationship is consistent with the previous discussion. Higher average lengths of stay yield significantly higher average occupancy rates, and states with larger hospitals (generally more densely populated states) also have significantly higher average occupancy rates. These variables are quite significant and explain a surprisingly large proportion of the variation in occupancy rates.

Conclusions

Empirical observations on the performance of the hospital sector are consistent with theoretical predictions. There appear to be many opportunities for reducing expenditures without making equivalent sacrifices in health care benefits, although it is difficult to estimate the magnitudes of the inefficiencies with any precision. My assessment of the existing literature on the relative sizes of the potential inefficiencies is the following. We can group potential efficiency losses into two categories—one reflecting distortions that lead hospitals to provide particular levels and patterns of care at other than minimum cost and the other reflecting distortions associated with excessive quantities and intensities of care. Then the losses from non-cost-minimizing behavior are small relative to the losses associated with consumption distortions and associated supply-side responses to satisfy excessive demands for services. The critical question is whether one or more of these targets of opportunity can be captured without making individuals worse off (in an ex ante utility-maximizing sense) using the policy instruments at our disposal.

4   A Framework for Evaluating Alternative Regulatory Mechanisms

A variety of schemes for improving the efficiency of the hospital sector and for controlling hospital costs have been suggested. Of the specific regulatory instruments used by state regulatory commissions for several years, those that have attracted the most attention fall into two broad categories. The first is certificate-of-need (CON) regulation. These regulatory programs seek to use hospital facility planning and permitting authority to control the construction of new hospital facilities and the renovation or alteration of existing hospital facilities. Building a new hospital, expanding an old hospital, or providing a new service must meet specific criteria established by state law and be approved by a state regulatory agency. This form of regulatory constraint is most often applied when the expected capital expenditures for a new facility exceed some threshold value. The objectives that a CON agency might pursue and implementation of CON regulations determine the effects of this regulatory scheme on resource allocation to and within the hospital sector.

A second regulatory approach to perceived problems of resource misallocation in the hospital sector involves controls over reimbursement. This form of economic regulation involves regulatory approval of an individual hospital's posted charges, the terms of reimbursement under cost-based third-party reimbursement contracts, and the total revenues that it can generate in any year. This type of regulation is sometimes referred to as rate regulation, making an implicit analogy with price regulation in regulated industries such as electric, gas, and telephone utilities. I prefer to refer to this general form of regulation as reimbursement regulation. With traditional public utility price regulation, the prices charged determine the demand for services and associated welfare losses arising from prices that are not equal to the marginal cost of service. In contrast, effective reimbursement regulation must be designed to affect the supply decisions of the hospital and does not alter directly the incentives to demand care.

Alternative models of both CON regulation and reimbursement regulation that I develop below share one characteristic: they are designed to affect the supply of hospital care directly. They affect the demand for care either not at all or only indirectly. These regulatory mechanisms are not aimed at changing the explicit terms of the insurance contracts between patients and third-party payers. For example, these regulatory instruments do not directly affect the deductible and coinsurance provisions of insurance contracts or the broad categories of service that are covered. Rather, they are aimed at affecting the incentives of hospitals to supply particular quantities and qualities of care as well as their financial incentives to supply all care that is demanded. In the best of all worlds these instruments induce hospitals to provide existing levels of care at lower unit costs or to ration the demand for care so that care with low expected benefits relative to costs would not be supplied. To the extent that the latter can be accomplished effectively, hospitals inevitably get into an ex post excess demand situation, and the implicit terms of insurance contracts are in fact altered. However, by eliminating resource expenditures associated with moral hazard, at least in principle, the reductions in a patient's freedom to consume hospital care are ex ante more than compensated for by a reduction in insurance premiums.

It is useful to evaluate the variants of CON regulation and reimbursement regulation using a common set of criteria. The evaluation criteria must themselves be based on the underlying sources of resource misallocation in the hospital sector and must consider the costs of using the regulatory alternatives.

Evaluation Criteria

One way of thinking about regulatory solutions is in terms of a search for institutional arrangements that allow us to simulate ideal insurance contracts. If it were not for moral hazard problems (demand responses by insured patients and associated supply responses by providers), supply-side distortions induced by low coinsurance rates, and agency problems, the ideal insurance policy would provide complete insurance. From a regulatory perspective, the issue is whether we can create institutions that can effectively reduce moral hazard problems, eliminate supply-side distortions, and reduce agency problems without incurring additional costs that offset the gains. No single instrument need do all these things, but can some instruments be found that can reduce indicated efficiency losses without sacrificing more than is saved?

In evaluating alternative regulatory instruments, I assume that basic provisions of the prevailing contractual relationships between individuals and their insurers remain the same. The system is assumed to continue to be characterized by virtually complete insurance coverage in the sense that the patient's out-of-pocket expense for all care provided represents a tiny fraction of the cost of that care. In other words, the consumption incentive that individual consumers face as a result of prevailing insurance contracts remains unchanged, and patient demands for care associated with this incentive are unchanged. Regulatory initiatives are viewed as affecting the supply side of the system directly by constraining the ability of hospitals to provide particular services at particular volumes (through certificate-of-need type regulations) or indirectly by affecting the ways in which providers are reimbursed for supplying care (reimbursement regulation). The analysis of the alternative supply-side regulations is then conducted in the context of performance characteristics associated with each regulatory instrument.

The following performance characteristics are considered. They reflect the potential sources of resource misallocation discussed and the economic and political characteristics of the individual instruments themselves.

1. Duplication of facilities and exploitation of Scale Economies. Does a particular regulatory instrument constrain the system's tendency to provide too many facilities offering similar diagnostic and therapeutic services given the ways in which the unit costs of care vary with the volume of care provided in a particular facility and taking the demand for care as given?

For facility duplication to be a problem, specific diagnostic and therapeutic services (such as CT scanners or open-heart surgery facilities) must be characterized by increasing returns (economies of scale) over some range of output. Quality competition between hospitals is presumed to lead to more facilities than would be indicated by a comparison of the cost characteristics of the facility and the demand for services. For example, assume that the cost characteristics of CT scanners are such that unit costs are minimized at 3,000 patient procedures per year. A health service area should have no more than one such facility if aggregate demand is less than or equal to 3,000 patient procedures per year. If the area has two facilities each performing 1,500 patient procedures per year, one of these facilities is a candidate for consolidation, reducing unit costs of providing CT scans in this service area.

Actual computations involving facility duplication are complicated by the costs of patients' traveling longer distances to a facility. In addition, in less densely populated areas demand may not be sufficient to achieve all scale economies or even to allow a facility to break even if reimbursement is based on average unit cost.[1] A demand that is insufficient to exploit all scale economies does not necessarily imply that the facility should not be built. In certain circumstances a subsidy might even be desirable if average cost pricing would not make the facility economical.[2]

Note that this inquiry takes prevailing levels of demand and patterns of care as given and asks whether these services can be provided more economically with a smaller number of facilities.[3]

2. Consumption Inefficiencies. Here we are concerned with the moral hazard problem. Even the optimal insurance policy (as opposed to the ideal insurance policy) is likely to lead us to observe ex post consumption behavior characterized, on the margin, by expected benefits substantially below costs, because of inherent difficulties insurers have in enforcing appropriate ex post levels of care while preserving the risk-spreading benefits of insurance. These kinds of problems are compounded by tax incentives and government programs that lead the system to provide overly extensive insurance contracts. Are there regulatory instruments that can restrict the provision of care characterized by unfavorable cost-benefit ratios?

3. Organizational Slack. We identified two interrelated reasons to believe that hospitals may be characterized by organizational slack, or x-inefficiency. Virtually complete insurance tends to eliminate price competition among providers. Without price competition the market has no independent natural selection mechanisms to eliminate inefficient providers. The prevalence of nonprofit hospitals which cannot be assumed to be cost minimizers compounds this problem. Does a particular regulatory mechanism provide incentives to hospitals to minimize the costs of production by eliminating organizational slack, or x-inefficiency?

4. Rate of Product Innovation. There are several reasons to believe that the rate of product innovation is too high. Low coinsurance rates tend to increase the rate of utilization of any particular technology beyond the point at which expected benefits equal expected costs. Duplication of hospital facilities increases the number of facilities purchased by hospitals even more. Tax incentives to purchase insurance policies that are too complete

expand the demand for new diagnostic and therapeutic services even further. Assuming that the rate of product innovation is at least partially influenced by the expected size of the market for a new technique, we can expect these considerations to lead to a rate of product innovation that is too high. Do specific regulatory instruments directly or indirectly tend to reduce the rate of product innovation?

5. Process Innovations. A dynamic analogue of organizational slack or x-efficiency is a bias against process innovations, that is, cost-reducing innovations in diagnostic or therapeutic techniques. By reinforcing cost-minimizing incentives, can regulatory instruments increase the incentives to develop and introduce process innovations?

6. Agency Problems. Ideally, we expect physicians to act as perfect agents for patients, given their health care problems and their insurance contracts. We encounter an agency problem if physicians recommend the provision of medical resources that are not beneficial (absolutely or compared with alternatives) or provide benefits smaller than the out-of-pocket costs to the insured patient. On the other hand, we expect physicians to recommend all the care that has expected benefits greater than the out-of-pocket costs to the patient, maximizing the individual's welfare after he becomes ill. We do not ordinarily expect physicians to act as perfect agents for society, making decisions so as to maximize ex ante utility.[4]

Perhaps this is a narrow notion of the agency problem, but I think it is useful. To the extent that physicians apply diagnostic or therapeutic techniques having zero or negative benefits, the physician is not acting as a perfect agent for either the patient or society. It is in this context that the agency problem is normally defined. However, the physician who acts as a perfect agent for the insured patient, applying medical resources beyond the point where benefits and costs are equal on the margin, may be acting in the best interests of the insured patient but not in the best interests of society. The physician in a sense facilitates the moral hazard problem by acting in the best interests of the insured patient. The ideal physician-agent does not create the moral hazard problem but helps the insured patient to exploit fully the incentives of the insurance system. To the extent that physicians tend to prescribe more care than would maximize the welfare of the patient, given the low coinsurance rate, can we devise regulatory mechanisms that constrain such behavior, increasing consumer welfare in both an ex ante and an ex post sense?

7. Excess Demand for Care. We expect the unconstrained hospital system to be characterized by an equilibrium that equates supply and demand. Health status, demographic characteristics of the population, and the characteristics of insurance packages determined the demand for care. Under the cost-based or charge-based reimbursement system, hospitals have strong incentives to supply all the demand. We have assumed that the explicit nature of the contractual relationship between patients and insurers is unchanged by regulation. This implies (excluding agency problems) that the latent demand for care by patients is unchanged. The regulatory instruments considered all operate on the supply side, providing either direct restrictions on supply behavior by hospitals or indirect restrictions by changing reimbursement and altering supply incentives. Supply-side responses that reduce unit costs without affecting the capacity of the system to deliver care will not disturb the balance between supply and demand in any fundamental way. However, instruments that reduce the aggregate capacity of the hospital system to provide various types of care will engender excess demand. If and when excess demand emerges, we must be ready to deal with the question of allocating the scarce resources. To the extent that available supplies can be directed to their highest-valued uses, moral hazard problems may be reduced and consumer welfare increased.[5]

Available capacity could be rationed by hospitals and physicians in a variety of ways. Available resources might be allocated to their highest-valued uses. Some demand would go unsatisfied, but it would be the care that is valued less than the effective shadow price of care implied by the supply constraint. In an ordinary market faced with a supply constraint, we would expect prices to rise and decentralized market forces to direct the available resources to their highest-valued uses. This is unlikely to happen in the hospital sector. Instead, hospitals will have to develop internal administrative mechanisms to allocate scarce resources, mechanisms that do not now exist because the insurance-reimbursement system signals all agents that resources are virtually free. How will hospitals allocate resources if supply constraints are imposed? How will patients evaluate a system that apparently gives them entitlements to free care but does not have the resources to provide it? We do not really know the answer to either question, but we can inquire into the tendency of any of the proposed regulatory instruments to create excess demand, and we can speculate about how it might be rationalized and how it will be perceived by patients.

The tax subsidies to insurance complicate this situation even further. If we choose to view as distortions the incentives that tax subsidies give to consumers to purchase even more complete insurance, then regulatory constraints that attempt to counteract fully the tax distortions would run into serious public acceptance problems. In this case effective supply constraints could lead to such large implicit restrictions on insurance contracts that the after-tax reduction in insurance premiums would be too small to compensate for the reduction in benefits. That is, given the tax subsidies, consumers would not purchase this type of contract even if it were made available by the market. Tax subsidies essentially increase the willingness to pay for a given level of care, and regulatory initiatives that try to counteract this tax-induced increase in demand will conflict with the individual's perceived ex ante and ex post welfare.

All these problems emerge even if we assume that a regulatory agency can determine the right amount of hospital capacity. In addition, the regulatory authority may be too stringent, slowing the rate of introduction of new technologies below optimal levels and restricting the ultimate availability of diagnostic and treatment facilities. Although the public interest rationale for regulation is based on the perception that the unconstrained system provides too much care, stringent regulatory constraints could move the system too far in the other direction. In much the same way as the Food and Drug Administration[6] appears to have slowed the rate of introduction of new drugs too much by using a stringent efficacy standard, the application of similar standards or arbitrary utilization and expenditure growth criteria could lead to similar results for hospital care. A system characterized by welfare losses resulting from supplying "too much" care may be replaced by a system supplying "too little" care or an undesirable distribution of care.

The terms *excess demand* and *rationing* almost inevitibly lead to pictures of a system that leaves large numbers of patients uncared for, leaves people dying in the streets, and generally involves repeated decisions regarding who shall live and who shall die. A system with such very severe supply constraints is an extreme that the American hospital system need not come to by making significant improvements in resource allocation. Excess demand and how it might be rationed is of considerable importance in evaluating alternative regulatory mechanisms, however. It is therefore worth considering further the excess demand problem and the associated rationing problems that regulators are likely to face before we proceed to discuss the remaining evaluation criteria.

In an ordinary competitive market demand and supply are brought into balance by commodity prices. How much of a particular commodity is consumed and how this consumption is distributed among consumers depends on willingness and ability to pay for service and on the costs of providing those services. Absent price controls, there is no excess demand, and supply and demand are rationed by prices. Prevailing insurance and reimbursement institutions have minimized the role of prices in determining the allocation of resources to and within the hospital system. Aside from time costs and the disutility of visiting a physician or spending time in a hospital, the out-of-pocket cost of hospitalization for most individuals is only a tiny fraction of the real resource cost. What patients demand is primarily a function of their perceived medical needs, their perceptions about what medical science can do for them, and the treatment deemed necessary by their physicians. Prices and incomes play a relatively small role in determining the patient-physician demand for services for most insured individuals. Under prevailing reimbursement systems virtually all demands are supplied. As a result, the value of care, on the margin, is probably quite low.

Let us examine the components of the demand for services. The process of want formation for hospital services is necessarily complex. The typical patient has little direct demand for hospital services. He feels that he requires medical attention and sees a physician for advice. (In more and more cases he goes to a hospital outpatient clinic or the emergency room.) The physician examines the patient and determines the most appropriate of the alternative treatments. Medical science is not anywhere near the stage at which one can scientifically define the "best" course of treatment in all circumstances. For a particular medical problem one physician may recommend medical treatment on an outpatient basis, another physician may recommend inpatient medical treatment, a third physician may recommend prompt surgery on an inpatient basis, and a fourth may recommend surgery on an outpatient basis.

Depending on the medical problem and the range of therapeutic alternatives, there may be a wide range of recommendations with essentially indistinguishable differences in expected benefits but perhaps substantial differences in expected resource costs. In the absence of cost considerations, physicians may recommend different treatments based on their own understanding of the patient and his problem, their experience with different therapies, and the weights they put on what is often conflicting scientific evidence. Thus in many situations, but certainly not all, "optimal" medical practice may be consistent with a variety of therapies.

This diversity extends to the specific implementation of a course of treatment once a patient is admitted to the hospital as well. Some physicians may feel that it is best to continue hospitalization for, say, a week. Another physician may feel that five days is sufficient and that the potential for contracting a disease while in the hospital or the risk of additional tests and treatments outweighs any additional medical benefits of a longer stay. There are wide interregional and intercountry differences in length of stay, surgical rates, and modes of treatment, often with no evidence that one course of action provides clearly better expected benefits to the patient. These differences reflect continuing differences in modes of practice for delivering the optimal medical care.

A physician may also develop a whole range of alternative courses of treatment. He may believe that some are better for the patient than others but that the inferior modes of treatment are better than nothing. We can think of a whole array of alternatives that provide different expected benefits from the viewpoint of either an individual physician or the medical community. Of course, if cost is not relevant to the decision, the physician will choose the mode of care he thinks is best. In this case, treatments that fall outside the broad ranges of best medical practice would not be chosen by well-informed physicians.

Thus, even in a system without resource constraints, we should expect to see considerable diversity, given the nature of medical science. However, this diversity will be bounded and will not generally include modes of care that, although better than nothing, are considered suboptimal.

In a system in which the costs of care are a relevant decision variable, we would expect a number of things to happen. First, we would expect much greater use of the lowest-cost alternatives. If there is little to recommend one course of treatment over another on medical grounds, cost becomes an important decision variable. For example, if in many cases there is little scientific basis to choose between inpatient and outpatient tonsillectomy, outpatient surgery might become the preferred alternative if it costs less. Similarly, if there is little scientific evidence indicating that a seven-day stay is better than a six-day stay, we would get shorter lengths of stay to conserve on resource expenditures. In these cases there appear to be opportunities to conserve resources with little or no distinguishable difference in the expected outcomes for the patient.

Much more problematical are situations in which there is a clear dividing line between the expected benefits of alternative treatments. Medical treatment of angina may make life more tolerable for a patient, but open-heart surgery may be the optimal treatment in terms of patient benefits. A patient with a coronary condition may be better served by being in an ordinary medical unit in a hospital than at home, but still better served by being in an intensive care unit. A patient with a concussion may be well served by a general examination by a physician, but still better served, perhaps only marginally, by having a CT scan as well. At the extreme a patient with kidney failure can survive for many years with kidney dialysis but would die without it. When we extend our range to allow for real differences in the quality of care, taking costs into account means that difficult cost-benefit decisions must be made. It is precisely these "tragic choices" that a system without supply constraints allows us to avoid.

When we begin to talk about supply constraints and the need to ration care to satisfy the constraint imposed by the availability of scarce resources, we are talking not about a single type of rationing decision but about a continuum. Relatively modest supply constraints could in principle be accomplished with very little sacrifice in health care benefits if this constraint could be met primarily by shifting to more cost-effective procedures. As we tighten the constraint, we gradually move from cost-effectiveness decisions to cost-benefit decisions. But given the current situation, we should expect to find many cost-saving alternatives that require fairly small sacrifices in benefits. As we tighten the constraint further, we naturally face more profound trade-offs between cost and quality.

Suppose that with a supply constraint, we could be sure that demands for care would be rationed efficiently. That is, the constraint would first be met by choosing among effectively equal courses of treatment on cost-effectiveness grounds, and low-valued increments in quality would be off next. Then we should expect that fairly substantial resource savings could be achieved without requiring very large sacrifices of patients.[7] After all, the issue is that a primary source of misallocation in the present system is the tendency to provide all care that is even marginally beneficial. Presumably, significant resource constraints could in theory be accommodated by increasing cost effectiveness and reducing the quality of care a little bit on the margin.

Even in an ideal world our ability to conserve resources while sacrificing very little depends on the size of the supply constraint. However, at this point we have no way of knowing precisely how the rationing will take place in practice. Hospitals and physicians have become accustomed to ignoring costs. As a result we have developed no accepted mechanism for nonprice rationing. Even a modest resource constraint could impose large sacrifices on patients, could be administered inequitably, and could rapidly confront substantial political opposition if rationing does not take place by exploiting opportunities to increase cost effectiveness and by gradually "moving up" the demand function. Although the opportunities for trading off large cost savings against small or insignificant benefit sacrifices has a certain theoretical appeal, we must ask how rationing might take place in practice.

We have relatively little to guide us, since this type of rationing does not generally take place in our hospital system. We can briefly examine the experiences of the HMOs, which implicitly face supply constraints, as well as the experience of the British National Health system, which is a supply-constrained system.

Although our understanding of the behavior and performance of HMOs in the United States remains fairly limited, some emerging trends are worth noting. Luft provides an excellent summary of the available evidence concerning how HMOs achieve their cost savings.[8] The primary difference between approximately comparable populations is a substantial reduction in hospitalization for HMO enrollees. A variety of forms of outpatient care are apparently substituted for hospitalization, but the net cost savings seem to be substantial. How much of this shift is due to provider incentives and how much is due to the elimination of patient incentives to seek hospitalization is unclear. We have even less information about the treatments provided to hospitalized patients. There appears to be little difference in average length of stay between hospitalized HMO enrollees and control groups. Therefore it appears that the admission decision is the primary rationing instrument. The use of specific hospitals by HMOs or the use of HMO-owned and operated hospitals in the case of Kaiser may allow HMOs to admit patients to less costly facilities and to have more control over the availability and utilization of specific services. However, there is no evidence that HMO enrollment has any significant positive or negative effects on broad measures of health status. Unfortunately, the evidence on the behavior and performance of HMOs is too limited to draw detailed conclusions. In addition, the available evidence is tainted by self-selection biases, other noncomparabilities in the comparison population, and the undocumented utilization of out-of-plan services. However, HMO enrollees are normally free to choose an alternative insurance scheme if the HMO provides inadequate services. Thus the success of a few HMOs provides a fairly strong indication that supply constraints of some magnitude can be accommodated by changing patterns of care without significant reductions in the quality of care. It also indicates that these savings can be accomplished without government regulation.

The British National Health System (NHS) offers (almost) free care to the entire population. Because it is a nationalized system, however, the capabilities of the hospital sector to deliver care depend on the resources allocated by the government. There is general agreement that the NHS is a severely supply-constrained system. Cooper provides a detailed discussion and critique of how these scarce resources are rationed by the NHS.[9] The system imposes long queues for hospital admissions (on the order of 15 weeks on average). In addition, he notes that certain valuable therapies such as dialysis, optimal treatments for hemophilic patients, and heart operations for children are sharply constrained by the lack of resources while therapies that do not appear to be cost effective are provided to others. Culyer raises serious questions about the mechanisms for queuing patients for hospital admissions and the general failure of the system to develop useful criteria for insuring that patients who most need prompt hospital care get it first.[10] Many commentators have also noted substantial regional variations in the resource availability and waiting times for hospital admissions. Furthermore, those in the upper classes appear to be able to gain access to the system more easily than those from the lower classes. Thus, faced with the need to ration care, the NHS has developed a rationing system that is far from optimal on either efficiency or equity grounds. Although the population has generally been satisfied with the performance of the system, dissatisfaction appears to be increasing, especially among younger patients with higher expectations than their elders. The NHS has spent over 30 years refining and reorganizing the system in an effort to improve the distribution of resources throughout the country and to different levels of the health system as well as the use of crude queuing systems to ration care. As Culyer's discussion indicates, this is not an easy task.

An inevitable conflict here exists between what might be accomplished in theory and what is likely to result in practice when binding exogenous supply constraints are placed on the hospital system. On the one hand, there appear to be abundant opportunities to alter patterns of care in order to save resources without imposing substantial sacrifices on patients. There are also substantial opportunities to trade off the quality of care against the cost of care; these opportunities raise more difficult allocational problems. However, drawing a demand function and conceptualizing a rationing scheme in which we eliminate low-valued uses first and then gradually move up the value function until the supply constraint is met is far easier than devising a rationing system that can do this efficiently and fairly, especially if physicians face limited incentives to do so. The HMO experience indicates that this can be accomplished to some extent by creating institutions with appropriate incentives to compete with other delivery systems. The NHS experience indicates that centralized supply constraints combined with considerable physician freedom can lead to rationing schemes that are far from ideal in terms of either efficiency or equity.

There is also the question of how insured patients will view a system that does not provide all the care they would otherwise demand, given the consumption incentives provided by their insurance contracts. Let us ignore tax distortions for the moment. In this case, to the extent that a regulatory instrument can reduce moral hazard problems by efficiently constraining the provision of low-valued care, the reduction in insurance premiums resulting from the associated reduction in hospital expenditures should more than compensate for the implicit restrictions that now become inherent in the insurance contract. Faced with the choice of a high-priced insurance package without these restrictions and a low-priced insurance package with them, the "typical" individual (but not necessarily every individual) would choose the second contract (which for some reason the unregulated market is not providing). Once the insured individual becomes ill, however, his financial incentives to demand care are still influenced primarily by the deductible and coinsurance provisions of his insurance contract. By accepting the contract he may have implicitly promised to be willing to forego care that has low expected benefits— even if, based on his costs as a result of his insurance, he would choose to have it. After the fact, he is still likely to want all the care he can have, constrained only by the direct financial costs and not by the implicit promises of the initial contract. Patients may object strenuously to perceived restrictions on the care that hospitals are willing to provide, since that care will be allocated by administrative rules rather than by price. Complaints about queues and the difficulty in gaining hospital admission are frequent among members of HMOs and are problems in systems with severe supply constraints like the National Health System in England.

How much patients object to such ex post restrictions no doubt depends on the perceptions of the benefits sacrificed,[11] their understanding of the actual entitlements of their insurance contracts,[12] the way in which hospitals allocate scarce health care resources among individuals, and whether they have freely chosen the restricted contract or had it imposed on them by the government.

Clearly, considerations of excess demand and associated rationing schemes must be an important criterion for evaluating alternative regulatory mechanisms. On the one hand, since the regulatory mechanisms that I will be considering achieve their effects by changing the supply side of the system and since excessive consumption accounts for the bulk of the inefficiencies, effective regulation is likely to require that supply will fall short of demand. On the other hand, a system that does not lead to efficient rationing of the associated excess demand may be very costly and politically unacceptable.

8. Potential Effects on Hospital Expenditures. The primary political motivation for government regulation of the hospital sector is the reduction of the level and growth rate of expenditures in

the sector. While expenditure behavior and consumer welfare are unlikely to be identical, we must at least inquire about the prospects of alternative regulatory mechanisms for achieving narrow expenditure goals. This is one of the few variables that we will be able to observe directly and fairly consistently. We will often have to be satisfied with using such data to draw inferences about the effects of different regulatory constraints. If regulation is successful in satisfying any of the first seven criteria, this should be observable in the expenditure data.

9. Information and Administrative Costs. Any regulatory system needs information about the structure, behavior, and performance of the system to help formulate rules and regulations for constraining it. Similarly, the application of particular regulatory instruments will entail administrative costs incurred by both regulatory agencies and providers. In evaluating alternative regulatory mechanisms, we want to know the kinds of information needed to achieve the objectives of the regulations and how much it will cost to obtain the relevant information. We also want to know the magnitude of the administrative costs incurred by government agencies and providers. Information and administrative costs are real costs to society and must be factored into any evaluative calculus. Furthermore, a careful analysis of the kinds of information needed to formulate sensible regulations and the costs of applying and enforcing them should give useful insights into how alternative regulatory instruments will actually perform compared with what they are supposed to do. No matter how good a particular regulatory scheme looks in theory, it will always perform less than perfectly in practice. Since information and enforcement costs appear to play a critical role in the failure of the private insurance system to offer "ideal" insurance contracts, we must ask whether government agencies are likely to be better able to obtain the relevant information and to enforce more efficient demand and supply behavior than are private agents such as Blue Cross.

10. Regulatory Distortions. The use of administrative regulation may simultaneously lead to responsive firm or industry behavior with undesirable efficiency characteristics. Thus rate-of-return regulation of public utilities may lead them to depart from cost-minimizing production behavior as they continue to seek to maximize profits in the face of a regulatory constraint.[13] In this case the welfare benefits resulting from regulatory successes in reducing

prices may be partially offset by supply-side distortions.[14] In evaluating hospital regulation, we must also consider the possibility that the instruments used may engender distortions on the demand or supply sides that at least partially offset the apparent gains from using these instruments.

11. Equity Considerations. Many of the institutions that characterize the ways in which individuals pay for health care and the ways in which health care is supplied are motivated by concerns about particular groups in society, primarily the poor and the elderly. In evaluating the performance of particular regulatory mechanisms, we should ask how these groups are likely to fare as a result of their application. We should also inquire whether the effects of alternative regulatory instruments will differ by region and for rural versus urban residents. These factors will play an important role in determining our ability to obtain the political consensus to implement regulatory programs that change the present system as well as affect the long-run viability of regulatory alternatives.

Conclusions

The first eight evaluation criteria follow directly from the discussion of potential market distortions, market imperfections, and associated categories of resource misallocation discussed in chapter 3. These "targets" for regulatory correction can be grouped into two categories: regulatory efforts to increase the efficiency with which prevailing levels of hospital services are provided, thereby reducing the unit costs of delivering that care, and regulatory efforts to constrain the quantity and quality of care supplied when the expected benefits of that care are lower than the costs of providing it.

These two foci of regulatory attention can be illustrated with the help of a simple diagram that considers only the static efficiency losses at issue. Figure 4.1 presents aggregate demand and supply functions for hospital admissions in a typical health service area at a point in time. S_A represents the actual marginal and average costs of providing care under current institutional arrangements. It includes any excess costs resulting from the hospital sector's tendency to depart from cost-minimizing supply (organizational slack, duplication of facilities). S_O represents the marginal and average costs of supplying care at minimum cost.

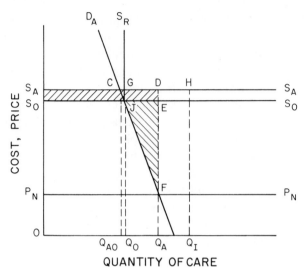

Figure 4.1 Demand and Supply of Hospital Care

S_O is drawn below S_A since any inefficiencies inherent in the current supply situation are assumed to be eliminated in drawing S_O. D_A represents the demand for hospital admissions given any particular net price of care confronted by the insured patient. The net price reflects only the proportion of actual hospital costs that the patient must pay for out-of-pocket plus the patient's opportunity costs of spending time in the hospital. The line P_N gives the net price of care at any particular level of hospital admissions given the associated costs of providing that care and any opportunity costs that affect demand. For simplicity it is drawn here as a constant fraction of the actual unit costs of providing hospital care given by S_A.

   In an unregulated system the net price of care is given by P_N, and the demand for care is given by Q_A. All care demanded is supplied at unit cost given by S_A. It is clear that on the margin the net price of care and the value of that care is less than the marginal cost of supplying it. There are two sources of inefficiency in this stylized system. First, with Q_A given, the unit cost of supplying care is higher than it would be if care were supplied at minimum cost. The difference in the expenditures per admission associated with this type of inefficiency is given by the line segment DE. The extra expenditures incurred as a result of this inefficiency are given by the hatched rectangle $S_A DES_O$ (total expenditures are given by the larger rectangle $S_A DQ_A O$). Second, taking the current costs of care as given (S_A), we see that all care consumed beyond Q_{AO} has a cost that is greater than its value to the individuals admitted since curve D_A reflects the willingness to pay for different qualities of care and beyond Q_{AO} it lies below S_A. The efficiency loss associated with providing this additional care is given by the hatched triangle *CDF*. Note, however, that this loss due to moral hazard may be optimal in the second best sense discussed in chapter 3. We can be assured that controlling this moral hazard improves the situation only if there are not offsetting losses in the risk-spreading characteristics of the insurance package (or offsetting transactions costs) that are greater than any ex post efficiency gains. Additional expenditures on care beyond Q_{AO} are given by CDQ_AQ_{AO}. As the figure is drawn here, these additional expenditures amount to about 40 percent of the total expenditures, although the welfare loss associated with providing this care carries a considerably smaller valuation. While expenditure reductions associated with moving from S_A to S_O are approximately equal to the efficiency or welfare loss, changes in expenditures associated with consumption inefficiencies are not appropriate measures of welfare losses. Welfare losses due to moral hazard generally have a value that is less than the actual expenditures associated with providing this care and depend on how flat the demand function gets beyond Q_O. This result emerges because the care provided beyond Q_O still has value, even though the value may be less than the costs of providing it.

The figure also indicates that efforts to capture efficiency losses associated with departures from cost-minimizing behavior by the hospital sector need not lead to nonprice rationing of demand (excess demand for care). As the figure is drawn here, if regulatory initiatives could promote greater supply efficiency, prevailing levels of care could simply be provided at lower cost. Indeed, reducing unit costs from S_A to S_O would decrease the net price of care slightly and increase equilibrium demand for care. On the other hand, reducing the amount of care supplied below Q_{AO} or Q_O requires that we impose a supply constraint that induces hospitals or physicians to ration care. Regulatory constraints that can induce this type of behavior must be represented as some type of capacity constraint on the supply of care. Such a constraint is represented by a vertical line S_R in figure 4.1. S_R represents the constrained capacity of the system to deliver care. It is drawn precisely at Q_O only for convenience and to represent the "optimal" supply constraint. We can think of S_R as a rule that says only Q_O admissions will be allowed, or a set of restrictions on the construction of hospital capacity to supply more care than is represented by Q_O, or perhaps a budget constraint that allows hospitals to spend a fixed amount.

This type of supply constraint has several limitations. First, since in reality we know the location of the relevant supply and demand functions only with great uncertainty, it is extremely difficult to know where to place the appropriate level for S_R. Even in a simple static world this would be difficult. In the true dynamic context of hospital demand and supply it is impossible to locate the "right" constraint with any precision. Second, this constraint simply operates on supply; it does not provide any guidance for rationing demand appropriately. We can only hope that the lowest-valued uses, represented by the portion of the demand function beyond Q_O, are rationed out. However, there is no way, a priori, to be sure that the rationing will actually be done this way. By setting S_R incorrectly, or if there is a scheme that rations high-valued uses rather than low-valued uses, we can easily reduce the effectiveness of a regulatory constraint or even make the allocation of resources to and within the hospital sector worse than the status quo.

We can also consider agency problems in the context of this simple diagram. Agency problems involve the provision of care that has no value to the patient or has a value so small that it is even less than the typical patient's net cost of care. Agency problems emerge either because of ignorance on the part of physicians and hospitals or because of conscious decisions to provide excessive care in pursuit of provider objectives rather than patient welfare. We have characterized this type of agency problem by denoting a point Q_I on the diagram. The difference between Q_I and Q_A represents the consumption of provider-induced care that patients would not take if they were well informed. The additional expenditures associated with the provision of such care are almost pure waste since the value of that care is negligible, zero, or perhaps even negative. As with the supply of care associated with moral hazard problems, supply-side constraints do not necessarily provide any direct mechanism for rationing these types of treatment. It is of course hoped that providing supply-side constraints, whatever rationing mechanism emerges, will first eliminate care that provides essentially no benefits.

This simple static characterization indicates the nature of the targets for regulatory attention, measurement issues, and some of the problems inherent in constraining what may be the most important sources of resource misallocation. This is only a simple stylized picture of the issues discussed. In particular no effort has been made to incorporate technological change and shifting demand for care resulting from changes in the size and demographic composition of the population and increases in per capita incomes. Introducing these characteristics does not change the basic qualitative analysis presented but does complicate the issues analytically and, perhaps more important, in terms of practical implementation.

Nor does this diagram address the last three evaluation criteria. Any theoretical gains associated with any particular regulatory instrument must be evaluated in the context of administrative costs, undesirable regulatory distortions, and the distributional consequences of the regulatory intervention. Administrative costs and costly regulatory distortions must be subtracted from any theoretical savings identified. An otherwise effective regulatory system that conflicts with basic distributional objectives and general criteria of fairness and equity is unlikely to obtain the political consensus necessary for implementation or long-run viability.

Certificate-of-Need Regulation

Supply-side regulatory interventions that directly constrain the ability of hospitals to add, expand, or renovate facilities require individual hospitals to obtain a permit when the associated investment expenditures exceed some threshold value. Hospitals must satisfy some set of need criteria to make the desired capital expenditures. This type of regulatory constraint on capital investment is embodied in the certificate-of-need process. Forty-eight states now have certificate-of-need programs. The investment threshold is normally $100,000 or $150,000.[1] These programs have been supplemented by voluntary agreements between the states and the federal government under section 1122 of the Social Security Act whereby the federal government can deny reimbursement to hospitals under federal programs if facilities have not been approved by a health systems agency (HSA) established under PL 93-641.[2] In addition, Blue Cross plans in some states will not reimburse for facilities that have not been approved by HSAs.[3]

Historical Background: Comprehensive Planning

Certificate-of-need regulation grew out of local, state, and federal efforts at comprehensive planning for the provision of hospital facilities. Certificate-of-need regulation continues to be closely interrelated with a very complex local, state, and federal planning apparatus.[4]

Local efforts at health planning go back at least to the early 1930s. At that time hospitals were heavily dependent on philanthropic contributions to pay for new facilities. Joint fund-raising efforts in many communities naturally led to questions of how the scarce capital resources should be allocated among the many competing "needs" for them. To help organizations allocate funds and to convince corporate contributors that funds were needed and were being wisely used, several cities created independent agencies to plan hospital facilities.[5]

The development of a facility-planning apparatus was given considerable impetus with the passage of the Hospital Survey and

Construction Act of 1946 (Hill-Burton). The Hill-Burton Act was a response to a perceived shortage of hospital facilities and a poor distribution resulting from limited funding for new construction during the depression and World War II. The need for more funding was also related to rapid improvements in medical science that were occurring at about the same time.[6] The Hill-Burton Act provided funds to survey hospital needs in each state, followed by grants to the state to carry out construction programs approved by designated state agencies and by the federal government. In the early years Hill-Burton programs focused on bed needs and the expansion of the stock of general hospital beds, using fairly rigid quantitative criteria for need.[7] The development of criteria at the federal level and the allocation of funds to states was not characterized by extensive cooperation or interaction between state and federal governments. There was apparently little federal interest in expanding state and local health-planning capabilities. In later years funding priorities changed,[8] and in the early 1960s the Hill-Burton program began to allocate funds to encourage the development of area-wide planning agencies. These autonomous local or regional agencies received grants from the federal government, but there was little federal control over what they did, and no necessary connections with related state agencies.

Local and state planning agencies were concerned with developing plans that seemed to establish priorities for the use of available funds. The planning agencies were not concerned with cost control, nor apparently was the federal government. It was also clearly in the interest of the hospitals to become closely involved with local and state planning efforts to avail themselves of federal funds to the maximum extent.

In 1966 the Comprehensive Health Planning Act (CHP) was signed into law. The act provided modest funding for the creation of an agency within each state with the responsibility for organizing the state's health-planning activities and for approving federal grants to area-wide planning councils. The state agencies were called the A agencies, and the local agencies were called the B agencies. The local agencies had to find at least half of their funding from local sources and came to rely heavily on hospitals for such funding. Not surprisingly there were very close working relationships between the B agencies and the local hospitals.[9] Although no reference is made to the specific organizational structure of these agencies in the statute, federal administrators decided that these agencies should be controlled by consumers and required that a majority of the members of each agency's governing council be consumers rather than providers. In conjunction with local planning efforts the CHP agencies also had a role in reviewing and commenting on federal funding proposals within their areas.

The 1966 act was a triumph of organizational complexity over substance. Federal funding and direction for the agencies was minimal, and the goals of the agencies were poorly articulated. There was little real interest in Congress or the Department of Health, Education, and Welfare in area-wide planning at this time.[10] Cost containment was not a major goal of the federal program, and the CHP agencies had little power over hospital supply decisions, except to the extent that they could influence the allocation of Hill-Burton funds or Public Health Service funds. With the growth of private insurance coverage during the previous decade, dependence on federal grants was declining. Yet the 1966 act created a comprehensive planning ethos and organizational structure for comprehensive planning based on interest group politics, a structure that has greatly influenced subsequent developments in both planning and facility regulation. The early evolution of this and related programs placed hospitals in the general posture of supporting comprehensive planning efforts. I suspect that at this early stage their interest was in securing as much federal money as they could and protecting themselves from the diversion of federal funds to other hospitals or other types of providers.[11]

The interest in using the planning agencies as vehicles for constraining the expansion of hospital facilities and increases in hospital costs, at least at the federal level, seems to have begun in earnest after the introduction of the Medicare and Medicaid programs. These programs led to a tremendous expansion in the demand for hospital care by the elderly and the poor, and federal and state government expenditures on hospitals increased rapidly. Hospitals had a new source of cost-based third-party payment to help finance expansion, renovation, and the introduction of new diagnostic and therapeutic techniques. Section 1122 of the Social Security Amendments of 1972 provided that capital costs associated with federal reimbursement for Medicare, Medicaid, and certain other federal programs could be denied if not approved by the state-designated planning agency. The states could voluntarily agree with the federal government to have a designated state agency review projects with capital costs greater than $100,000. If approval was not attained, the federal government could then deny reimbursement for the interest and depreciation associated with such a project and allocated to Medicaid patients. Since in general this would amount to a trivial proportion of the total costs of such a project,[12] it is unlikely that in and of itself this requirement could have represented a substantial disincentive to hospitals.[13] Unlike a formal certificate-of-need agency, hospitals could proceed with or without CHP agency approval even in states that had review agreements with the federal government. Of more importance is that many Blue Cross plans began to require CHP agency approval for hospitals to obtain reimbursement for expenditures associated with a particular facility.[14]

The National Health Planning and Resource Development Act of 1974 (PL 93-641) is the latest federal effort to encourage health planning at the state and local levels. This act is clearly much more concerned with issues of unnecessary facility construction and escalating health care costs. The law creates a national network of health systems agencies (HSAs), which are required to collect and analyze data related to health planning, establish health system plans in their areas (HSPs), develop annual implementation plans (AIPs), make recommendations to a designated state agency on the need for new facilities and the appropriateness of existing facilities, and allocate federal funds within their areas. The act provides federal funds for the HSAs, which may be private non-profit corporations or public agencies. As with the old B agencies, all interest groups must be represented on governing boards, a majority of whose members must be consumers. The HSAs cannot accept funding from health care providers, however.

In addition to the area-wide HSAs, the act provides for the creation of a state health planning and development agency (a government agency) and a state health coordinating council (public and private representatives). The state health coordinating council is to review and coordinate the activities of the HSAs, review the state's overall health plan, and approve the disposition of federal funds allocated to the states. The health planning and development agencies were to prepare state health plans based on the HSA plans and to administer a certificate-of-need program. (If this all sounds very complicated, be assured that it is.)

Perhaps the most important requirement of the new planning law was that the states had to establish certificate-of-need programs meeting certain minimum criteria[15] or else sacrifice certain federal funds.[16] Certificate-of-need programs were therefore embedded both conceptually and legally into the comprehensive planning process. They provided the real "teeth" for a process that had evolved from one initially designed to expand capacity to one designed to constrain a system that would otherwise provide more capacity than would be desirable. Recent amendments to the 1974 act have exempted HMOs from certain certificate-of-need requirements and have encouraged state and local agencies to promote competition where it can work effectively.[17]

The 1974 act represents a much more serious effort on the part of the federal government to influence state and local hospital supply decisions while maintaining at least the appearance of a decentralized system sensitive to local conditions and concerns. Federal funding has been increased, dependence on local hospitals for funding has been eliminated, and federal agencies now take a much greater hand in establishing guidelines to be used to evaluate the need for specific facilities[18] and the development of minimal criteria for state certificate-of-need agencies.[19] The act reflects the increasing federal and state concern with the costs of Medicare and Medicaid and the view that comprehensive planning plus certificate-of-need regulation could make a major contribution to controlling increases in hospital expenditures without reducing the quality of care available to the population.

Theoretical Considerations

The concept of need is necessarily ambiguous. In the following discussion I develop two different models of certificate-of-need agency objectives. The first model (CON1) focuses primarily on facility duplication. The notion is that the hospital system tends to supply any particular level of demand at other than minimum cost because more hospitals offer specific services in any health service area than are economically efficient. The efficiency loss is due primarily to a failure to exploit economies of scale. In the context of figure 4.1 CON1 represents an effort to increase the efficiency with which hospital care is supplied by reducing S_A. Since a major source of facility duplication is nonprice competition among hospitals, CON1 may be viewed as representing objectives similar to those of a hospital cartel.[20] However, independent hospital objectives to offer a wide range of services implies that the objectives implicit in CON1 and the interests of the hospitals do not completely coincide.[21]

The facility duplication problem is depicted graphically in figure 5.1. Let's assume that we are focusing on open-heart surgery facilities and that over some range of utilization these facilities are characterized by decreasing average costs. Let's say that two hospitals in proximity to one another both offer this service with annual utilization rates of q_1 and q_2 respectively. If all these patients were treated in a single facility ($q_1 + q_2$), scale economies would be more fully exploited and the total cost of providing these services would decline. We are taking demand as given; if only one hospital offered the service, the total volume of open-heart procedures in this area would not change. In this conceptualization of certificate-of-need regulation, only one facility would be able to obtain a permit unless it could be shown that the area-wide demand was high enough to allow a second facility to exploit fully scale economies as well. To the extent that facility duplication of this type can be constrained, we have a clear welfare gain. Demand is unaffected, but the costs of delivering care are reduced. There may be additional benefits associated with establishing minimum annual volumes for particular facilities that are related to medical efficacy rather than production cost.[22]

This simple conceptualization of CON regulation requires that the regulatory agency establish utilization criteria for applications to add or renovate facilities. To establish such criteria requires information on facility cost functions and on current and expected

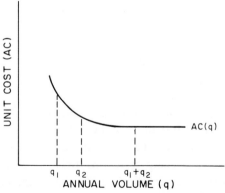

Figure 5.1 Variation of Unit Cost with Volume for a Hypothetical Facility

demand in terms of both aggregate volumes and patient locations. The regulatory agency must not only examine "technical" economies of scale but also consider the patients' additional travel costs. Even if a particular facility is not fully exploiting all technical scale economies, the costs of transporting patients over longer distances will at some point outweigh the savings in unit production costs. These costs involve ordinary travel costs as well as sacrifices in the quality of care associated with imposing longer treatment delays on trauma patients. Distance is of special concern when evaluating facilities in areas of low population density where demands are unlikely to be large enough to exploit all available scale economies. The federal government has promulgated facility guidelines for several categories of facility.[23] Individual state commissions have sometimes promulgated their own guidelines.[24] Until fairly recently the major focus was on the supply of general hospital beds.[25]

The overall effects of this type of certificate-of-need process on potential inefficiencies in the hospital sector and on total hospital expenditures are likely to be fairly small, for a number of reasons.

1. This type of regulation focuses directly on only one of the many potential performance failures of the hospital sector—facility duplication. Since demand is taken as given, this type of regulation essentially endeavors to reorganize the system so that available scale economies are better exploited. The basic quantities and intensities of care do not change. Schwartz and Joskow have evaluated the theoretical savings that might be achieved via consolidations consistent with federal guidelines in four areas that have attracted considerable attention.[26] They conclude that the anticipated savings, ignoring administrative costs and implementation difficulties, represent a small fraction of total hospital expenditures and that such consolidations can accomplish only a small fraction of the administration's cost containment goals. Since CON regulation operates on the margin, it may take a long time to achieve even these savings.

Indirect effects of certificate-of-need regulation may be worth considering. First, reducing the number of facilities reduces the market for new diagnostic and therapeutic techniques. To the extent that efforts to develop new products are related to the anticipated size of the market, the rate of product innovation may be reduced. This indirect effect is difficult to quantify, and the disincentives associated with a smaller U.S. market are attenuated by the international availability of many of these techniques. As a result, it is almost certainly insignificant.

Second, the CON agency may use its formal authority to consider applications for new or expanded facilities to extend its authority beyond the boundaries of the statute. For example, a hospital applying to build a new ten-bed intensive care unit may be told (informally) that the application will be approved only if it closes its obstetrical unit or agrees to provide expanded outpatient facilities that would reduce inpatient utilization. How far a CON agency can legally go in creating an informal regulatory process based on informal bargaining between the regulatory staff and the applicant is unclear. However, these types of informal regulatory processes have evolved in other regulated industries,[27] and there is some evidence that it has become an important component of the certificate-of-need process in some states.[28]

2. By establishing fairly high threshold capital expenditures to trigger CON review, the CON process covers only a fraction of the decisions that a hospital makes every year. Furthermore, by focusing regulation on a particular input—capital—the process may ignore some of the most costly supply decisions that hospitals make and induce costly input substitutions of labor and materials for capital. Hospitals are not particularly capital intensive. Interest and depreciation expenses account for only about 10 percent of total hospital expenditure, and there is no simple relationship between the capital expenditures associated with making a particular service available and the total costs of that service.[29] Where there are substitution possibilities between capital and other inputs, CON regulation may encourage the introduction of less capital intensive but more expensive ways of making particular services available.

The implicit assumption underlying most discussions of certificate-of-need regulation is that hospital services are characterized by a production function with fixed proportions of capital, labor, and materials per unit of output. There is no reason to believe that this assumption is valid. Indeed, there appear to be large opportunities for input substitution. As a result, providers are likely to respond to a constraint on only one input by using other inputs more intensively. At best, this reduces the impact of CON regulation; at worst, it can actually increase the costs of providing services.

3. The establishment of utilization criteria may create perverse incentives for hospitals and physicians to increase the utilization of particular services beyond what would otherwise be desirable in order to satisfy the guidelines.[30] If one believes that agency problems are important, this kind of distortion must also be considered.

4. Havighurst[31] and others have suggested that it may be fairly easy for existing hospitals with substantial political power to "capture" this process. Thus new hospitals or freestanding facilities may find it difficult to enter the market when it means that their entry will make it difficult for existing hospitals to expand their own facilities or when the effects of increased competition will be undesirable from the perspective of existing providers. To the extent that new entrants such as HMOs or freestanding clinics can provide services more efficiently, this restriction represents another potential distortion in the system. A related problem is the prospect that large and powerful urban teaching hospitals will be able to exploit this process at the expense of smaller and less powerful rural and suburban hospitals. The real or perceived equity properties of this system may be quite unattractive.

5. The information costs and administrative costs of a CON process of this type are likely to be quite high. Since the process requires that individual hospitals obtain permits to build new facilities, renovate existing facilities, and in some cases merely change the uses of existing facilities, CON involves a large number of case-by-case determinations based on general utilization criteria and specific criteria applied to individual applications. Both the agency and the providers must spend time and money preparing and reviewing applications and engaging in administrative and judicial procedures. Case-by-case determination may also impose long lags on the construction of new facilities. The more extensive the CON agencies' authority to review hospital facilities, the more expensive this process becomes.

Overall, I expect this form of CON regulation to be successful in reducing the most egregious departures from minimum cost production associated with facility duplication. The opportunities for cost saving, however, are relatively small and are further reduced by the administrative costs of such regulations as well as by potential distortions that the system might generate. It would not be surprising to find that vigorous CON programs have significant effects on the supply of beds and the number of diagnostic and therapeutic facilities without having a substantial effect on total hospital expenditure.[32]

The second conceptualization of the CON process (CON2) allows the certificate-of-need agency to have a much broader perspective of need. Here the agency recognizes not only that facility duplication produces inefficiencies but also that in some ideal sense the quantity and quality of care is too high. CON regulation is viewed here as trying to do more than reorganize the system to supply prevailing demand levels more efficiently. This type of agency also tries to use its authority to place a binding supply constraint on the system. The capital-constraint strategy tries to restrict the ability of hospitals to expand their capacity, *even if* facility expansion is accomplished at minimum efficient scale. In the context of figure 4.1 CON2 endeavors to use capacity constraints to establish S_R at some level below Q_A. The intent is to use capital constraints both to force the system to exploit fully available scale economies and to enforce supply constraints that ration prevailing levels of demand.

Early versions of the Carter administration's cost containment legislation included a national ceiling on annual capital expenditures, which would have been allocated among the states according to a variety of characteristics, in the first year by population. Essentially, the capital constraint would have given the state CON agencies a budget constraint limiting the total amount of capital expenditures that they could approve.[33]

This model of CON agency objectives reflects a concern about consumption inefficiencies as well as supply inefficiencies associated with facility duplication.[34] The idea is not just that there are too many CT scanners to satisfy demand efficiently but that too many patients are being provided with CT scans. Thus the CON process can be viewed as trying to force the system to generate appropriate levels of care by constraining supply. Supply is constrained in turn by restricting the amount of capital that can be used to produce hospital services. From figure 4.1 and previous chapters we can see that at least in theory, this conceptualization of CON authority has much greater opportunities to reduce expenditures and improve the allocation of resources because it affects both the unit costs of care and the capacity of the system to deliver care.

This type of regulatory objective places much greater burdens than CON1 on both the regulatory agencies and the hospitals. To implement a capital-constraint scheme such as this, the CON agency needs the same kinds of information required to implement the less restrictive objectives of CON1. In addition, the agency must make decisions about the capacity for performing diagnostic and therapeutic techniques relative to the anticipated demand for that capacity. To do this efficiently, it must determine costs and benefits on the margin for many types of facilities located in many different communities. Assuming that it could establish the "right" amount of capacity, it then must rely on hospitals to allocate the available resources to their highest-valued uses. Hospitals are not now organized to make such trade-offs,[35] and this regulatory strategy provides no independent incentives for patients or physicians to accommodate reduced supply with concomitant reductions in the demand for care having the lowest expected benefits. Furthermore, biasing the supply constraints to facilities that the CON agency can control and focusing only on capital rather than providing a general resource constraint may also distort hospital responses in many ways. Ideally, hospitals would have to develop some internal rationing mechanism for allocating available resources to their highest-valued uses. Placing constraints on a single input satisfying some lower-bound threshold will limit the ability of hospitals to do so.

The information requirements for implementing this strategy are enormous. The CON agency is essentially trying to reduce the moral hazard problem by restricting the amount of care available. It tries to do this by approving only enough aggregate supply to provide an "appropriate" aggregate level of care. The agency hopes that the hospitals can ration the excess demand efficiently. Furthermore, the CON agency must try to do this with control only over capital rather than over total expenditures. Even the control over the capital input is incomplete because of the relatively high threshold capital expenditure level that has been established. Reducing the threshold increases the difficulty of the CON agency's task enormously because it begins to encompass too many specific expenditure decisions that are part of a very complex hospital supply system. The process is also subject to political maneuvering and extensive litigation by both hospitals and individual communities. With the broader constraints implicit in the CON2 model, the stakes increase beyond the number of facilities needed to satisfy demand efficiently to the ultimate question of the aggregate amount and quality of care available in a state or community. Those without significant political power are much more likely to be disadvantaged by a system such as this.

Absent federal constraints on capital expenditures by the individual states, it is hard to imagine that state CON agencies would independently turn to the more restrictive notion of need. The benefits of such a strategy—lower insurance premiums—are likely to be diffuse and difficult to perceive by local consumers. Although it is conceivable that in the long run everyone would be better off with a system that constrained care whose expected benefits are far below its costs (lower premiums and more complete insurance with less moral hazard), individual patients and communities are likely to perceive the sacrifices much more quickly and directly than the benefits. The elderly, with entitlements through Medicare, will not see the benefits. Individual communities will not see their Blue Cross rates reduced in response to individual restrictions placed on them. Medicaid beneficiaries will see only that their access to care has been reduced. Without freedom to choose among different plans and with the real or imagined inequities that administrative allocation of resources by government agencies and hospital organizations entails, this "strong" model of certificate-of-need is not likely to characterize most CON agencies. Most CON agencies do not have direct cost-control responsibilities or broader controls on reimbursement policies. Without any real budget constraint and faced with broad objectives covering both need and efficiency, such agencies are likely to be susceptible to provider and community pressures, especially when a reasonable case can be made that the quantity and quality of care available in the community will be reduced significantly.

As long as the constraints applied by CON agencies are not too severe and focus attention primarily on duplication in a relatively small set of facility categories, the approach is probably workable. However, when we recognize the relatively small theoretical savings that can be achieved by focusing on facility duplication, the administrative costs of regulation, and "exceptions" engendered by interest group politics, the gains to be expected from this type of regulation are probably small. To the extent that the process discourages the entry or expansion of more efficient providers and engenders perverse supply-side responses, the savings will be reduced even further. As a result, it is not surprising that hospitals have not vigorously opposed and have even encouraged the introduction of weak certificate-of-need constraints.

Nor should it be surprising that the federal government has taken an interest in giving CON agencies (as opposed to the hospitals themselves) capital budget constraints limiting the aggregate amount of hospital investment that they can approve. Without such a constraint or independent responsibilities for hospital costs, CON agencies are likely to constrain expenditures that engender minimal community and hospital opposition. The apparent simplicity of the capital budget approach is very misleading, however. A constraint low enough to have significant effects on hospital capacity will probably create excess demand problems. Once we adopt such a rationing mode, we no longer have an administrative process that is simple in either theory or practice. To the extent that patients and their physicians value the services that can no longer be made available, the process could quickly become an administrative and political nightmare, with competing interests vying for the available resources and with the regulatory agency having no direct way to compensate those who believe that their health care benefits have been reduced.[36] We should not hope that the certificate-of-need process can do more than implied by the first model of the process' objectives. Indeed, it would probably be undesirable to try to use such a process for more than constraining the most obvious cases of facility duplication, because of the inherent limitations of this regulatory strategy. Table 5.1 summarizes the expected effects of CON1 and CON2 in terms of the eleven evaluation criteria identified in chapter 4.

The Diffusion of Certificate-of-Need Regulation

Interest in establishing some form of regulatory control on the expansion of hospital facilities at the state level preceded the passage of federal comprehensive planning legislation in 1966 but quickly became entangled with it. Curran argues that serious attention to public control of health care facilities began in 1959 with a series of meetings between the U.S. Public Health Service and the American Hospital Association[37] and was motivated by the first major denial of a Blue Cross rate increase by a state insurance commission. New York was the first state to enact a certificate-of-need law, the 1964 Metcalf-McCloskey Act. The act was passed in response to a legislative study of hospital costs and health insurance rates. The law provided for controls of new facilities and the expansion of old ones and established the criterion of

Table 5.1 Performance of Two Models of Certificate-of-Need Objectives

Criterion	CON1	CON2
1. Facility Duplication	Potentially effective	Potentially effective
2. Consumption Inefficiencies	Not effective	Potentially effective
3. Organizational Slack	Not effective	Not effective
4. Rate of Product Innovation	Not effective	Potentially effective
5. Process Innovations	Not effective, possibly perverse	Not effective, possibly perverse
6. Agency Problems	Not effective, possibly perverse	Potentially effective
7. Rationing Care	Not effective	Potentially effective, possibly perverse
8. Expenditure Effects	Small	Potentially large
9. Information and Administrative Costs	Large	Very large
10. Regulatory Distortions	Likely	Likely
11. Equity Considerations	Modest potential for problems	Large potential for problems

public need. This early initiative in New York contained most of the essential features of the certificate-of-need laws that have now spread to other states.

Who supported such laws? In many cases they were supported by state and local health planning agencies, insurance companies, and hospital associations.[38] As Medicare and Medicaid expenditures began to increase rapidly, federal and state interest in these laws increased as well. Much has been made of the support given to comprehensive planning and certificate-of-need laws by the American Hospital Association (AHA) and often by state hospital associations. The AHA would have supported such legislation, for a variety of reasons. First, as Curran has suggested, the hospitals, represented by the AHA, saw that regulation was coming and decided to support it so that they could affect the way it proceeded and perhaps structure the regulatory process to keep it from damaging their interests. Earlier participation in local planning under Hill-Burton, and even before, should have convinced the hospitals that they could have substantial influence if the process could be structured so that they could dominate it. Second, Havighurst has suggested that the hospitals viewed the certificate-of-need process from a "private interest" perspective[39] as repre-

senting a cartelizing device that would restrict the system's tendencies to generate excess capacity by restricting new entrants
and "excessive" competition. There is probably something to this,
but the "private interest" and "public interest" rationales for some
supply restriction are likely to be similar and thus extremely difficult to distinguish.[40] While the AHA's support for comprehensive
planning was enthusiastic, its support for formal regulation was
much lower on the priority list.[41] The creation of a model bill and
active support for state certificate-of-need legislation by the AHA
in 1968 and 1969 was at least partially preemptive and, I believe,
partially a response to restrictions on Blue Cross rate increases by
state insurance commissions.

Hospital costs were increasing rapidly even before the introduction of Medicaid and Medicare, fueled largely by expanding
private insurance coverage by both Blue Cross and private insurance companies. In many states insurance commissions regulate
Blue Cross rates as well as the rates charged by private insurers.[42]
At least in theory, state insurance commissions can indirectly constrain hospital costs by denying insurance premium rate increases
on the grounds that the insurance carriers should have been more
diligent in monitoring hospital expenditures. However, with a
comprehensive planning and certificate-of-need process, all approved major facility programs would have the government stamp
on them and would by definition represent reasonable expenditures for which insurers correctly reimbursed. To the extent that
the hospitals could hope to get this approval without incurring
severe supply constraints, they may have viewed CON regulation,
first, as an attractive way of preempting efforts by state commissions to force insurance carriers to deny reimbursement for some
expenditures and, second, as a limitation on the ability of state
insurance commissions to restrict the flow of funds from third
parties into the hospital sector.

The AHA, along with government agencies and health insurers,
has by and large continued to support comprehensive planning
and enforcement mechanisms.[43] The AHA has opposed efforts to
increase federal authority and the imposition of federal need criteria on state and local agencies, however, and has lobbied actively
against the Carter administration's proposal to give state agencies
stringent capital expenditure constraints. The AHA's notion of
effective planning and facility regulation appears to be more consistent with the first model of the certificate-of-need process than

with the second model. When regulation becomes more stringent, opposition by state hospital associations has occurred.[44] The major opponents of CON-type regulation have been state medical societies (representing physicians) and proprietary hospitals.[45]

The link between area-wide planning and certificate-of-need regulation is a natural one. To make rational decisions about the number and distribution of hospital beds and diagnostic and therapeutic techniques requires detailed information about utilization patterns and costs. Criteria for need must be established, and some way for deciding among competing claims must be developed. Regulatory restrictions in the absence of a comprehensive plan based on the relevant demand and cost information are unlikely to lead to desirable results. Planning without regulatory restrictions is unlikely to have any effects. The peculiar parallel and often uncoordinated development of the local, state, and federal planning and regulatory apparatus has resulted in a plethora of agencies having both incomplete and overlapping authorities, often with inadequate funding to perform their mandates. This has almost certainly reduced the potential effectiveness of this system. Considerable rationalization and consolidation of agencies with planning authority and agencies with permit authority would certainly be desirable, and this seems to be occurring slowly.[46] Integration of this system with agencies having broader responsibilities for cost containment is also probably desirable.

Table 5.2 provides information on the status of CON authority in the individual states. The table indicates the year in which a certificate-of-need statute was enacted in each state and the year that a section 1122 agreement was signed. To be in conformity with PL 93-641 all states must have established a CON program meeting minimum federal criteria by the end of 1980.[47] Since 1122 programs are essentially redundant when a state has a CON program, many of them have been terminated.

By January 1980 all but three of the states had enacted certificate-of-need laws. Forty-three states had a section 1122 agreement with HEW at one time or another, although 16 of these have been or will be terminated.

Table 5.3 shows the diffusion pattern of CON legislation enacted by the states over time. Five states have had CON programs in operation for ten years or more, and another 21 states have had programs for at least five years. Thus the majority of states enacted

Table 5.2 Status of State Certificate-of-Need and Section 1122 Programs in the United States, 1980

State	Year CON Enacted	Section 1122 Agreement
Alabama	1977	Yes/modified
Alaska	1976	Yes
Arizona	1971	No
Arkansas	1975	Yes
California	1969	No
Colorado	1973	Terminated
Connecticut	1969	No
Delaware	1978	Yes
Florida	1972	Terminated
Georgia	1974	Yes
Hawaii	1974	Terminated
Idaho	—	Yes
Illinois	1974	Yes
Indiana	—	Yes
Iowa	1977	Yes
Kansas	1972	Yes
Kentucky	1972	Yes
Louisiana	—	Yes
Maine	1978	Yes
Maryland	1968	Terminated
Massachusetts	1971	No
Michigan	1972	Yes
Minnesota	1971	Yes
Missouri	1979	Yes
Mississippi	1979	Yes
Montana	1975	Yes
Nebraska	1979	Yes
Nevada	1971	Yes
New Hampshire	1979	Terminated
New Jersey	1971	Yes
New Mexico	1978	Yes
New York	1964	Terminated
North Carolina	1978	Yes
North Dakota	1971	Yes

Table 5.2 (continued)

State	Year CON Enacted	Section 1122 Agreement
Ohio	1975	Terminated
Oklahoma	1971	Yes
Oregon	1971	Terminated
Pennsylvania	1979	Terminated
Rhode Island	1968	No
South Carolina	1971	Yes
South Dakota	1972	No
Tennessee	1973	No
Texas	1975	No
Utah	1979	Terminated
Vermont	1979	Terminated
Virginia	1973	Terminated
Washington	1971	Yes
West Virginia	1977	Yes
Wisconsin	1977	Terminated
Wyoming	1977	Terminated

Source: U.S. Department of Health and Human Services.

Table 5.3 Number of States Introducing CON Regulation during Specific Time Periods

Period	Number of States
1964–1970	5
1971–1974	21
1975–1977	10
1978–1979	11
No program	3

Source: Table 5.2.

such programs before formal federal requirements were established and have been operating long enough to show some effects, if these agencies have been effective in constraining facility construction and hospital expenditures. It is probably not coincidental that four of the five states that enacted certificate-of-need laws before 1970 have also created state regulatory agencies to regulate hospital changes, reimbursement rates, or budgets.

At least superficially, state certificate-of-need programs are very similar to one another. All programs cover nursing homes and hospitals, while very few cover facilities in physician offices. The threshold level of capital expenditures that triggers a review is usually $150,000 (the federal standard) or $100,000. A few states have lower thresholds for equipment. CON programs are usually located in the state department of health. Here the similarities end, however, and there appear to be substantial practical differences in the orientation, procedures, and resources of CON programs.[48] The legislative mandates, monitoring and sanctions, real administrative resources, and the extent of development of review criteria vary enormously from state to state, and CON agency criteria may differ from HSA criteria.[49] The information and analyses that providers must submit vary considerably, as does the burden of proof. Also varying from state to state are interrelationships with other state agencies such as rate-setting commissions and HSA's, provider groups, and third-party payers. Perhaps most important, the general objectives and orientation of the programs vary. In some states the CON agencies are oriented primarily toward planning and certification procedures, while in other states they are oriented much more toward constraining the supply of facilities.[50] With so many differences in objectives, resources, and behavior, we should not be surprised to find large differences in the effects of the programs.

The CON program in Massachusetts is an interesting example of how such programs have evolved over time. A temporary CON law was passed by the state legislature in 1971 and made permanent in 1972. The CON law is administered by the Department of Public Health through the Public Health Council, which makes the decision on an application. The Public Health Council (PHC) consists of one full-time member, the commissioner of public health, who acts as chairman, and eight other members who are part-time volunteers serving essentially without compensation. Initially, the council operated without special funding or staff, drawing on the resources of the Department of Public Health. The council is now supported by a professional staff of about twelve with a budget of about $400,000 in the Determination of Need Office within the Department of Public Health. The PHC has jurisdiction over acute hospitals, nursing homes, and ambulatory care facilities. Hospitals must seek approval for projects involving capital expenditures of more than $150,000, the addition of four or more beds, or the introduction of a new service, even if the associated capital expenditures are below the threshold. Until late 1976 the council operated without any quantitative guidelines for evaluating need. Quantitative criteria for general hospital beds were not developed until late 1976, while quantitative criteria for other specific service facilities were not promulgated until 1978.[51]

Applicants denied approval by the council can appeal to the five-member Health Facilities Appeals Board. The unsuccessful applicant can then seek judicial review. In several instances unsuccessful applicants have appealed to the state legislature for special authorizing legislation overruling the CON decision. In the early years a few of these efforts were successful, but more recently such bills have either failed to receive legislative approval or have been vetoed by the governor.[52]

Over time, the analytical sophistication of the council staff and the requirements placed on applicants has increased. Indeed, the facility-specific criteria developed in Massachusetts have a much sounder analytical basis than those developed by the federal government. The council has gradually developed procedures to monitor the progress of projects that have been approved and now works closely with the state rate-setting commission. Although the CON program was established in 1972, it took several years to develop analytical capabilities and detailed quantitative criteria for evaluating projects.

As Bicknell and Walsh have demonstrated, the primary focus of the CON agency in the early years was on the supply of general hospital beds.[53] The council took a hard line on efforts to expand the supply of hospital beds, and it is in this area that applicants have had the most difficulty in obtaining approvals. During the period 1974–1977 bed-related projects in hospitals had an approval rate of 79 percent while other projects had an approval rate of over 95 percent.[54] Perhaps in response to the early emphasis on beds, more recent applications to expand the supply of general medical-surgical, pediatric, and obstetrical beds have declined to a trickle. Of 196 applications processed by the council between January 1975 and June 1979 less than 10 percent involved increases in the number of beds.[55] In all but a handful of cases, the applications were either denied or scaled back so that the total number of beds would not increase.[56] However, applications for new or expanded ancillary facilities have continued to increase and have an approval rate of over 95 percent. Beginning in 1976, the council began to take a harder line on new "high-technology" services such as CT scanners. Indeed, between 1977 and 1979 there was a virtual moratorium on approvals of new CT scanners in health service areas that already had one. However, over this period a large number of applications for new scanners were submitted (several were subsequently withdrawn), reflecting demands by hospitals for the latest technology and high utilization rates in existing facilities. Eight CT scanners were approved by the council in early 1979.

The applications that the CON agency must process vary enormously in terms of anticipated capital expenditures, type of services, and complexity of the issues. Table 5.4 provides more detailed information on the characteristics of CON applications that were decided in Massachusetts over the period 1975–1979. These applications involved capital expenditures that varied from essentially nothing to over $50 million and construction activities as mundane as the installation of a new boiler and as controversial as the construction of a new pediatric care facility.

The Massachusetts CON review process itself has been designed to assure participation by all those with an interest in the application. An application for a new facility is first submitted to the Determination of Need (DON) office within the Department of Public Health. The DON office reviews the application and is supposed to make a recommendation to the Public Health Council for final approval or denial within eight months. Copies of the application are also made available to the HSA in which the hospital is located, to the state rate-setting commission, and to the Office of State Health Planning. The HSA normally submits its own recommendation to the Public Health Council after reviewing the application and consulting with the DON office. The rate-setting commission and the State Office of Health Planning appear to play a primarily consultative role in support of the DON office's efforts to make a recommendation. DON recommendations and HSA recommendations occasionally differ, but this is very rare.

Table 5.4 Certificate-of-Need Decisions Involving Acute Hospital in Massachusetts, 1975–1979

Dates	New Equipment or Service		Replace Existing Equipment		Expand Existing Service		Clinic		Nonmedical Space or Equipment		Renovations	
	A	D	A	D	A	D	A	D	A	D	A	D
1/75 to 6/75	8	3	2	0	4	0	2	0	3	0	0	0
6/75 to 1/76	4	1	8	0	3	0	1	0	3	0	2	0
2/76 to 7/76	11	3	3	3	3	0	1	0	3	1	3	0
8/76 to 12/76	6	1	6	0	1	0	2	0	5	0	0	0
1/77 to 7/77	2	2	1	1	0	1	2	0	3	0	2	0
7/77 to 12/78	12	3	8	0	8	0	0	0	2	0	3	0
1/79 to 7/79	24	3	7	0	2	0	0	1	0	0	3	0
Totals	67	16	35	4	21	1	8	1	19	1	13	0

Source: Data collected from files of the Massachusetts Department of Public Health. Data do not include applications that were withdrawn prior to final determination.
A = approved.
D = denied.

In almost all cases the PHC approves the recommendation of the DON office. If an application is denied, the hospital can appeal or submit a revised application. In many cases resubmissions are eventually approved.

Crude approval-denial rates and associated capital expenditures are sometimes used as measures of CON agency effectiveness. However, approval rates are extremely poor measures of the effectiveness of any CON process, for several reasons. First, hospitals almost certainly adapt their applications to the rules, regulations, and ongoing decisions of the CON agency. If hospitals see, for example, that the CON agency has adopted stringent criteria for approving increases in the number of beds, then they may simply stop making such applications. Second, a substantial number of applications may simply be withdrawn without going through the entire process based on consultations with the CON agency's staff. Headen indicates that a significant fraction of the initial applications were subsequently withdrawn in Massachusetts.[57] On the other hand, hospitals may layer one application on another or continually resubmit applications in the hope that pressing the CON agency with additional applications will eventually lead the agency to approve some. In this case, a hospital may simply assume that it will not get all that it asks for and will ask for more than it expects. Finally, applications may be only partially approved or may be revised as the application goes through the review process.

Therefore, the approval-denial rates of different CON agencies do not really reveal the extent to which these agencies are deterring uneconomical expansion of hospital facilities. Even if the denials crudely represented the constraint that the CON agency placed on the hospitals under its jurisdiction, it would be incorrect to measure the "benefits" of the CON application by adding up the construction costs that have not been incurred as a result of the denials.[58] The construction costs of any facility are usually only a small fraction of the total costs that would be incurred by this facility if it were built and operated. Furthermore, if the facility is not built, patients who might have been treated there will probably be treated elsewhere, increasing the expenditures of neighboring facilities. The denial of the application may impose costs on patients served by the hospital in terms of longer travel times of lower-quality medical care. These costs must be subtracted in any benefit calculation. Finally, the CON application denied may lead to responses that cost even more as a result of the narrow "trigger" of capital expenditures that is used. Clearly a complete evaluation of the costs and benefits of CON regulation requires much more than this crude inquiry. The first step in a more thorough inquiry is to determine whether CON regulation is providing any measurable constraint on hospital facilities and hospital expenditures. If it is not, then this form of regulation cannot be having any effects on resource allocation. If there is evidence that CON agency activity reduces facility construction and hospital expenditures, we can then inquire into the social value of the constraints that have been observed.

My expectation is that the practical ability of CON agencies to constrain the expansion of facilities and the growth in expenditures will be extremely limited. This hypothesis is tested in chapter 7, which examines the available empirical evidence on the effects of state CON regulation in practice.

6 Government Regulation of Hospital Reimbursement

Certificate-of-need regulation, at least in theory, alters neither consumer incentives to demand care nor provider incentives to supply it. Instead it places a permit process between what hospitals would like to supply, given prevailing incentives, and what the law will allow them to supply. Final decisions about new facilities, which are captured by the CON net by virtue of the magnitude of their capital costs, are essentially shifted from the hospital to a regulatory agency. The likely performance characteristics of certificate-of-need regulation varies with the model chosen.

Supply-side constraints by administrative agencies need not take this form. We can think of an alternative regulatory system that alters the incentives of hospitals to supply various types and quantities of services. To effect hospital incentives while leaving patient incentives unaltered,[1] we essentially must intervene in the reimbursement system. As long as hospitals are assured of full reimbursement, they have no incentives to conserve resources and will supply all demand that is forthcoming.

It is therefore useful to consider efforts to regulate hospital charges, reimbursement rates, and budgets. Ideally such regulatory initiatives should strive to alter the incentives to supply care, to depart from cost-minimizing behavior, and to engage in uneconomic service rivalry and quality competition.

Historical Background

Hospital reimbursement regulation does not have the long tradition of the planning-CON process. Federal activity in this area has been limited to controls on hospital charges implemented as part of the Economic Stabilization Program in the early 1970s and certain restrictions on Medicare reimbursement rates established by regulations implementing section 223 of the Social Security Act Amendments of 1972. The Carter administration tried unsuccessfully to expand federal activity by establishing a cost containment program using budget constraints for individual hospitals. The program, had it been enacted by Congress, would have been a major step toward federal regulation of hospital expenditures and reimbursement rates.

In the absence of any comprehensive federal reimbursement regulatory program the creation of this type of regulatory process has been the result of state initiatives. A number of states had offices with certain types of reimbursement authority as early as the 1950s. However, these agencies were concerned primarily with establishing appropriate prices for hospital services purchased by the states on behalf of welfare recipients. They did not have broad hospital cost containment objectives.

State reimbursement regulation programs with broad cost containment objectives were generally developed after 1970. The creation of a state agency to collect cost and revenue data and to develop procedures for controlling hospital charges and budgets was often motivated by the burden of escalating Medicaid payments on state and local budgets and rapidly increasing Blue Cross premiums. In some states hospitals and insurers got together to form voluntary cost containment programs, at least in part to stave off formal state regulation. In other states Blue Cross plans began to experiment with alternative reimbursement formulas and reimbursement systems to help contain costs. By 1980 several states had established agencies to regulate hospital charges, reimbursement rates, or total hospital expenditures.[2] In addition, Blue Cross plans in several states have turned to detailed cost and reimbursement review programs that attempt to reimburse hospitals prospectively based on estimates of future costs and utilization patterns rather than retrospectively based on actual costs incurred by individual hospitals.[3] More recently New Jersey has begun an experiment in which hospitals are reimbursed a flat fee for particular medical problems.[4]

The Traditional Public Utility Model

States that chose to limit hospital expenditures by creating regulatory agencies with formal powers to constrain hospital charges and reimbursement rates needed some model on which to base their regulations. The earliest conceptualizations of reimbursement regulation seem to have been based on the public utility model of rate regulation.[5] The focus on traditional public utility regulation and associated ratemaking procedures and ratemaking rules was only natural. Almost all states had a long historical experience with this type of regulation and had developed fairly well defined procedures for regulating franchised natural monopolies. In its most rudimentary form we can think of state public utility regulation as being concerned primarily with two things.[6] First, at least in theory, they are supposed to ensure that franchised natural monopolies cannot exploit their monopoly power to charge monopoly prices and earn monopoly profits. Therefore one important aspect of public utility regulation is the determination of a fair rate of return on stockholders' investments and the application of this rate-of-return criterion to determine the total revenues that a firm can earn given its costs of production. Second, once the aggregate level of allowable revenues has been determined, the regulatory agency must establish appropriate rate structures.

The substantial research on state public utility regulation shows that this regulation has worked quite differently from what the simple theory might lead one to believe.[7] Nevertheless, in terms of basic economic principals and administrative procedure, this is the general framework in which regulation of franchised natural monopolies has taken place. By and large state public utility commissions have traditionally left decisions about how electricity (for example) would be produced and how much capacity would be available to the regulated monopolies themselves. Only egregious departures from prudent planning and production decisions encountered regulatory sanction. Furthermore, regulated natural monopolies have a legal obligation to serve all customers and to provide adequate service to these customers. In short, the direct efforts of state public utility commissions focuses primarily on profit regulation and rate structure determination, taking the costs incurred by firms as given except where such costs appeared unreasonable. One reason for this was a perception that profit-seeking utilities had independent incentives to supply service efficiently. A second reason was the recognition that the regulatory agency had insufficient expertise or information to evaluate most utility supply and production decisions. In recent years state agencies regulating electric utilities have become more interested in these supply-side decisions, but this interest seems to have caused more problems than it has solved.

The application of the public utility model of rate regulation to hospitals is problematical for several reasons.

1. The underlying problems that economic regulation of hospitals should be addressing are not primarily problems of potential

monopoly pricing and excessive profits resulting from a legal monopoly position. Applying traditional public utility principles to hospitals—insuring that prices and costs are approximately equal, allowing a fair rate of return on capital, assuming that firms by and large supply output at minimum cost and should plan to meet all demand at prevailing prices—does not deal with the fundamental sources of inefficiency and excessive expenditures in the hospital sector. We are not dealing with a natural monopoly problem here.

The basic problem is that expenditures keep increasing as a result of expanding utilization and increases in the intensity of care. The insurance system and its interaction with demographic changes and technological change lead to increases in demand. Hospitals have strong incentives to satisfy this demand, perhaps inefficiently, as long as they are assured of full reimbursement. The problem is not that prices are too high because of monopoly power. The problem is that demand is too high and that the costs of meeting that demand are too high. Just passing on the costs and ensuring that rates are high enough to allow the hospitals to satisfy all demand is not likely to be productive because this approach simply reinforces the incentives that led to the problem. In addition, nonprice competition and independent "rent-absorption" incentives of nonprofit hospitals are likely to ensure that any monopoly profits are dissipated by additional resource expenditures. Effective regulation of this type must focus on developing reimbursement constraints that encourage hospitals to satisfy demand at minimum cost and, more important, to ration demands that have low values relative to the costs of providing care.

Let me note one caveat to this general view. A hospital's ability in a monopolistically competitive market to price discriminate among services may enable it to use "profits" on some services to subsidize services that would otherwise be unsustainable. Ensuring that the charges for services are pegged closely to their costs may force a hospital to drop some services that are not self-sustaining. Unfortunately, it appears that services like emergency services and outpatient clinics would be most adversely affected by the elimination of cross-subsidization, and this may be an undesirable outcome from a variety of perspectives.[8]

2. Traditionally, monopoly prices distort consumer behavior because prices are greater than marginal cost. Demand is ineffi-

ciently constrained because prices are too high. The overwhelming majority of hospital patients do not see the posted charges since they have almost complete insurance coverage. Fiddling with the rate structures is not likely to affect the behavior of insured patients very much.[9] Demand is certainly not being overconstrained because prices are too high. It is the terms of reimbursement between third-party payers and hospitals and their effects on supply-side responses that are the most important targets for regulatory attention because of virtually complete insurance coverage.

3. The typical state public utility commission generally regulates a relatively small number of firms in any industry, and the products supplied by these firms are quite homogeneous. Electric utilities supply electricity and sell it to fairly homogeneous groups of residential, commercial, and industrial consumers. In contrast, the typical state has over a hundred acute hospitals that would fall under a regulatory agency's jurisdiction. These hospitals vary enormously by types of care provided and types of patients treated. Replacing reimbursement negotiation between providers and insurers with a public utilities–type regulatory scheme is likely to entail enormous increases in transactions costs. Hospital-by-hospital and service-by-service reimbursement regulation could easily become an administrative nightmare.

For rate regulation to have a significant effect on this system, we must go well beyond the traditional public utility model in which the objective is to match revenues with costs. Non-profit hospitals are likely to do this on their own. We must focus on the interaction between alternative reimbursement criteria and the incentives provided by different reimbursement formulas to supply care. We need normative criteria that focus on the "reasonableness" of the costs themselves rather than a complicated accounting exercise that tries to match posted prices (which are largely irrelevant here) with "actual" costs incurred.[10] The responses will depend largely on the criteria used to determine which expenditures are reimbursable and which are not. Much has been written on the virtues of prospective versus retrospective reimbursement.[11] This dichotomy in and of itself is not very important. The responses engendered by either system depend almost entirely on the criteria used to determine allowable expenditures and the importance of these criteria. Absent more detailed information on the reimbursement criteria, a prospective reimbursement system is not necessarily more constraining than a retrospective system.[12]

Alternative Reimbursement Criteria

A number of approaches for determining reimbursement have been suggested. I discuss three prototypes here, but variations or combinations are certainly possible.

1. The Comparable-Hospital Approach. The objective of this approach is to assemble data on sets of comparable hospitals, distinguish efficient from inefficient hospitals, and reimburse only for efficient costs.[13] Within each set, we compute the average expenditures per day or per service and then reimburse for no more than, say, the mean for the group. (Whether it is the mean or the median or the 80th percentile is not important here.) Hospitals with costs above the mean must either reduce their unit costs or run a loss. Hospitals below the mean get extra revenue, which they can spend as they see fit.

Another way of thinking about this procedure is to run a regression of unit costs (say per diem costs) against all relevant characteristics of hospitals for a large sample of hospitals.[14] These characteristics could include size, occupancy rate, patient mix, service offerings, teaching status, and average length of stay. We can then compare the actual costs for a hospital having certain characteristics with the predicted costs from the regression. The residuals distinguish the efficient from the inefficient. We might only allow reimbursement of predicted costs or predicted costs plus something. Hospitals above the regression line will be forced to reduce costs so that they approach the reimbursement standard, or else they will incur losses.[15]

With reference to the performance criteria developed in chapter 4 we can identify some strengths but many weaknesses of this approach used alone. This approach makes most sense in a static world where the major problem is that similar hospitals produce the same services with different levels of efficiency. It may be an effective way to deal with organizational slack and perhaps to encourage process innovations. However, a major characteristic of the hospital sector is that it is very dynamic. Expenditures increase with increases in utilization and intensity of care. There is no static production set or simple per diem or per illness cost function to anchor such a reimbursement process to. The characteristics used to group hospitals are precisely the factors that lead to increased expenditures. As a result, this approach alone is unlikely to affect the major dynamic elements of increasing hospital expenditures or the sources of inefficiency in the system.[16]

Even if the hospital sector were static, there is no reason to believe that the estimated cost function represents an efficient level of expenditure for each hospital. If we believe that all hospitals are offering care that is too resource intensive, tying all hospitals to the mean is not likely to deal effectively with the basic problem.

It appears that the generalized comparable-hospital approach will be effective primarily in reducing organizational slack and may encourage process innovations, since hospitals that can get below the cutoff point for their group can "keep" some of the cost savings and use the extra revenues for other purposes. However, the revenues could be used to accelerate the introduction of new diagnostic and therapeutic facilities. This approach seems unlikely to have a significant effect on facility duplication, especially if this is a general phenomenon, and it will not affect consumption inefficiencies, the rate of product innovation, or agency problems. There is no reason to believe that the approach will lead to the rationing of demand for care, since it is essentially a cost-plus procedure which corrects only for deviations from group norms. The overall potential for cost reduction of the comparable-hospital approach appears to be small.

Of course, the grouping of hospitals will determine the effects of this approach. I believe that the approach will almost inevitably lead to an ever-expanding set of relevant characteristics as individual hospitals argue that they are being unfairly treated because of differences in size, patient mix, service availabilies, teaching status, and so on. Thinking of this in a regression equation context, I fear that the characteristic set will expand until almost all interhospital cost variations are "explained." As the characteristic set expands, equity issues will gradually disappear, information costs will increase, and the effects on supply-side behavior will diminish. I believe that hospitals and their patients and physicians will find this procedure politically acceptable in the end, primarily because it can be easily manipulated to affect supply-side behavior very little. Therefore, in practice this scheme is unlikely to achieve even its limited potential.

2. Specific-Criterion Formulas. A second method for determining which expenditures should be reimbursed and which should not is to apply specific normative criteria on utilization rates for

entire hospitals or specific services within hospitals. For example, a regulatory agency may determine that general hospitals should have occupancy rates of at least 80 percent, obstetrical units occupancy rates of at least 65 percent, and pediatric units occupancy rates of at least 70 percent.[17] A hospital that has a utilization rate higher than the criterion is fully reimbursed for its costs. If it has a utilization level below the criterion, then its unit costs are recomputed to reflect what they would be if the criterion had been satisfied. The hospital is then reimbursed as if it satisfied the criterion.

As with the comparable hospital approach, hospitals whose costs are not fully reimbursed because they fail to meet the normative criterion must either achieve the criterion or find some way to subsidize the service. Assuming that cross-subsidization is not permitted, a hospital can respond in one of two ways. It may reduce supply, either by reducing its capacity to supply a particular service or by eliminating that service completely. Alternatively, it may try to meet the criterion by increasing utilization. Doctors may be encouraged to increase the average length of stay for inpatients or to treat more patients on an inpatient basis. The hospital may try to attract patients from neighboring facilities. Reducing supply is likely to reduce expenditures resulting from more thorough exploitation of economies of scale. Increasing utilization could actually increase expenditures.

This regulatory approach has many similarities to the first view of the certificate-of-need process. Specific utilization criteria for general hospital beds and specific services must be developed. In the CON process such criteria can be used to evaluate new capital expenditures over some specific size. Here the criteria are simply used to determine the extent to which costs are reimbursed. Both approaches have essentially the same performance characteristics, including the same relatively small prospects for expenditure savings. However, the use of reimbursement incentives instead of applying utilization or quantity criteria for approving the construction of new facilities has a number of potential advantages.

The CON process normally applies the criteria to new projects that require approval rather than to the existing stock of facilities (although informal negotiations may expand the de facto reach of certificate of need). Symmetrical reimbursement formulas can affect the entire stock of facilities and yield whatever additional economies of scale are to be had more quickly.

General reimbursement criteria will not have the tendency to discriminate against "new entrants" that may be able to produce specific services more efficiently than existing hospitals. It may also be more difficult for politically strong institutions to manipulate the system.

The combination of criterion reimbursement with data on comparable hospitals can provide incentives to eliminate organizational slack and to create better incentives for process innovations.

As with certificate-of-need regulation (at least the first model), the major savings to be expected from this approach arise from the elimination of facility duplication so that scale economies can be better exploited. Additional savings accrue from eliminating biases against new facilities relative to existing facilities. Combining utilization criteria with a comparable-cost formula may also help to eliminate organizational slack and create incentives for process innovations. However, the number of dimensions over which useful normative criteria can be specified (primarily regarding utilization rates) remains limited, and hospitals could respond perversely to these criteria by expanding utilization in a variety of ways.[18]

Once again, this regulatory approach deals primarily with static efficiency gains resulting from reductions in the unit costs of providing particular levels of care. It has little if any effect on the major causes of increases in hospital expenditures associated with overly high demands for care (in terms of quantity and intensity). Demand is not rationed; it is only reallocated so that it can be satisfied more efficiently.

3. General Budget Constraints. A third approach is to recognize that hospital expenditures are too high and growing too rapidly and simply to give hospitals a binding expenditure constraint below what they would incur if unconstrained. This is essentially the approach that the Carter administration tried to get Congress to take (without success).[19] For example, we might assume that unconstrained, real hospital expenditures will grow at 5 percent per year. The regulatory authorities somehow determine that this rate of growth is much too high and decide that a 1 percent real growth rate is "right." All hospitals are than told that they will be reimbursed in year t only for expenditures calculated according to the following formula:

$$E_t = E_{t-1} (1 + I + 0.01),$$

where E_t is the current year's expenditures, E_{t-1} is last year's expenditures, and I is an index of general inflation (percentage charge in input prices). This approach implicitly places restrictions on the growth in the quantity and intensity of care that can be supplied.

In terms of the performance criteria of chapter 4 this approach has a number of advantages over alternative efforts to control expenditures using administrative regulation. However, it also has a number of problems. Let's first discuss the advantages.

We get away from hospital-by-hospital and service-by-service cost and reimbursement regulation by applying a general budget constraint to all hospitals, yielding a regulatory process that is, on the surface, much less complex, arbitrary, and discriminatory.

We allow the individual hospitals to decide how their limited resources are to be spent rather than relying on regulators to specify utilization criteria for a laundry list of specific services. Since the "reach" of specific-service regulatory criteria is necessarily limited by the array and complexity of services provided, the general budget constraint extends the incentives to constrain expenditures over the full range of services offered by the hospitals and places the burden of establishing detailed normative criteria and internal resource allocation on those who best know the opportunity set and likely efficacy of care.

We provide incentives to eliminate organizational slack and to introduce process innovations.

We not only encourage static efficiency and process innovations but also constrain the hospital from expending resources on new product innovations and more intensive use of existing diagnostic and therapeutic techniques. By placing a binding budgetary constraint on hospitals, we simply do not allow them to provide the additional services demanded, which are the major source of increasing expenditures, without cutting back somewhere else. We force the system to ration the demands for hospital care.

We encourage changes in the internal organization of hospitals by forcing hospitals to develop internal mechanisms for allocating scarce resources so that they can ration demand. If done properly, these changes can reduce consumption inefficiencies or moral hazard problems.

At least in theory, general budget constraints get many good marks in terms of our performance criteria. Unfortunately, these theoretical advantages are offset by several practical disadvantages, some of which go to the heart of the "sustainability" of this type of regulatory system when superimposed on the prevailing insurance system. The disadvantages include the following.

A severe constraint on real increases in expenditures will almost inevitably lead to excess demand and nonprice rationing of demand. This regulatory strategy does not affect the economic incentives to demand more and better services; it only constrains the ability of hospitals to supply them. Neither the patient nor his physician has any additional incentives to conserve resources. The hospital will not be able to supply what is demanded and must ration demand. Rationing is a theoretical strength of this regulatory strategy, but it also raises practical problems of politics and equity. No matter how well the hospitals can allocate the available resources, patients are not likely to be satisfied with an insurance entitlement that promises "free" care but cannot supply it. The more binding the budget constraints, the more significant the resulting dissatisfactions of insured patients. This is especially true since the choice of the "right" growth rate in real expenditures is largely arbitrary, consumers are unlikely to perceive the benefits of such constraints in lower insurance premiums, and consumers are not free to choose among insurance plans with different implicit restrictions on benefits.

The simplicity of the general and uniform budgetary constraint that treats all hospitals equally is predicted on the implicit assumption that all hospitals should be treated equally. There is no reason to believe this. Hospitals differ as to the kinds of patients they serve, the base level of services offered (less sophisticated southern or rural hospitals would argue that they should be allowed to catch up to more sophisticated northern or urban hospitals), and a wide variety of teaching responsibilities. It is almost inevitable that a large proportion of hospitals will find plausible reasons for obtaining exceptions to the general formula.[20] Presumably some exceptions can be built into a simple formula, but a formal exception procedure would likely evolve. A conceptually simple regulatory instrument may quickly turn into a complex federal regulatory system with built-in aspects of the comparable-hospital and specific-criterion forms of reimbursement regulation.[21]

Since hospitals are not now organized to allocate scarce resources to their best uses, the rapid introduction of a severe budget constraint could easily lead to chaotic and arbitrary allocation rules which may be neither efficient nor perceived as being fair. This transitional problem can probably be avoided if the budget constraint is tightened gradually, giving hospitals sufficient time to adapt their internal processes for resource allocation to a binding budget constraint. However, even in the long run, I am skeptical about the willingness of different groups in society to accept hospital-established criteria for admissions and treatment. As with any supply-constrained system, some individuals will learn to use it to their advantage while others will be or will perceive that they have been locked out and are being discriminated against. Excess demand, combined with real or imagined inequalities in the decisions about who gets served, will inevitably lead to pressures to have the budget constraints relaxed.

As a practical matter, both the comparable-hospital and specific-criterion approaches may actually have some of the effects of a general binding budgetary constraint that explicitly restricts increases in volume and intensity as a result of regulatory lag. In an economy characterized by rapid inflation, regulatory lag can have profound effects on the behavior and performance of regulated firms.[22] Many of the state regulatory agencies with the authority to regulate hospital budgets and reimbursement rates incorporate some of the characteristics of the comparable-hospital approach.[23] After "reasonable" base-level costs have been determined, prospective budgets or rates are established using these base-level costs plus adjustments for anticipated increases in input prices and changes in volume and intensity.[24] To the extent that inflation is underestimated or changes in projected volume or intensity are less than they would be without a constraint, hospitals may find themselves facing much more stringent financial constraints than implied by the regulatory formula, at least between rate reviews. A not-so-subtle way of turning a weak reimbursement regulation process into one characterized by persistent binding budgetary constraints that affect more than departures from cost minimization is to consistently underestimate inflation and unconstrained changes in volume and intensity.[25] To the extent that regulatory lag is used in this way to turn less constraining forms of regulation into a general budget constraint system, we should observe strong pressures for retrospective adjustments for inflation and changes in volume and intensity if the administrative system is to account fully for them.

In light of the problems with stringent budget constraints, it is not surprising that Congress did not pass the cost containment legislation proposed by the Carter administration. Even if it had been passed, I suspect that it would have been quickly emasculated by exceptions, administrative complexity, and political pressures to relax the constraints. Hospitals are perceived to be spending too much money, so we pass a law requiring that they spend less. The process gives hospitals fiscal incentives to conserve resources but does not give similar incentives to the patient or the physician.

Not surprisingly, then, we face a dilemma. Regulatory initiatives that promise to yield the least in terms of efficiency gains and expenditure reduction encounter the fewest practical and political limitations. Those that promise to yield the most are likely to encounter the most severe political opposition and to require the most fundamental changes in hospital organization and behavior. The distortions that characterize the hospital sector are of two basic types: (1) Prevailing levels of care are provided at other than minimum cost. (2) The current system leads to demands for quantities and intensities of care that are too high; absent government intervention, supply will be expanded to satisfy these demands. By dealing with the first set of inefficiencies, we encounter no fundamental conflict between demand and supply. Unfortunately, we are not talking about a substantial fraction of current expenditures or the rate of growth in expenditures. When we try to deal with the second set of problems by constraining expansion to meet all demands, we inevitably thrust ourselves into a demand-supply conflict that is difficult to resolve without raising fundamental questions about the real meaning of the health care entitlements implicit in "complete" insurance contracts. If the individual consumer could see that he is better off with a much more restricted contract, the objections might be diminished. But the insured patient is unlikely to care much about any benefits from severe supply-side constraints that accrue ex ante. Without the freedom to choose among insurance plans with different contractual restrictions, the consumer may not perceive himself as being better off either. This problem is exacerbated because the linkages between the benefits of increased restrictions on taking care and perceived reductions in insurance premiums have been broken by tax subsidies, complete employer payment of premiums, and pervasive public programs that have no clear linkages between premiums and benefits.

The expected performance characteristics of the three reimbursement regulation schemes discussed in this chapter are summarized in table 6.1.

Mandatory State Reimbursement Regulation

By the end of 1980 eight states had active mandatory hospital rate regulation programs administered by a state agency (table 6.2). Colorado had such a program, but it was terminated in 1980. Several states have established rate review agencies, whose powers are largely advisory (table 6.3). As with state CON agencies, the institutional structure and methods used to regulate hospital rates vary enormously from state to state, and both the coverage and sophistication of these programs have increased over time. These formal state programs are supplemented by "voluntary" private rate review programs, generally implemented by Blue Cross plans, in 12 states (table 6.4).[26] However, I think that it is useful to distinguish formal state regulation of hospital reimbursement decisions from what amounts to a particular form of negotiation between major third-party payers and hospital providers. Blue Cross efforts in this area probably represent rational private market responses to enforce more efficient contracts between insurers and providers; they do not represent government intervention. The threat of state regulation may, however, make hospitals more receptive to alternative reimbursement arrangements with third-party payers.

Unlike planning and CON regulation, hospital associations have been much more cautious in their attitudes toward formal state regulation of hospital payments. They correctly view such legislation as having the potential to impose severe financial constraints on hospital behavior. They are especially concerned about rate review programs located in state or federal agencies, since the states and the federal government are the major third-party payers and may have strong incentives to severely restrict reimbursement rates. The hospital association in New York has expressed extreme dissatisfaction with the New York regulatory program because it has placed severe financial burdens on the hospitals.[27] Of course, this is exactly what a program that imposes severe budgetary constraints should be expected to do.

The state programs differ considerably in terms of organizational structure, methods of controlling reimbursement rates, types of

Table 6.1 Performance of Three Instruments for Regulating Hospital Reimbursement

Criterion	Comparable Hospital	Formula	General Budget Constraint
1. Facility duplication	Not effective	Potentially effective	Potentially effective
2. Consumption inefficiencies	Not effective	Not effective	Potentially effective
3. Organizational slack	Potentially effective	Not effective	Potentially effective
4. Rate of product innovation	Not effective	Not effective	Potentially effective
5. Process innovations	Potentially effective	Not effective	Potentially effective
6. Agency problems	Not effective	Not effective, possibly perverse	Potentially effective
7. Rationing care	Not effective	Not effective to moderately effective	Potentially effective
8. Expenditure effects	Small	Small	Potentially large
9. Information and administrative costs	Moderate	Large	Moderate
10. Regulatory distortions	Unlikely	Likely	Unlikely
11. Equity considerations	Little potential for problems	Modest potential for problems	Large potential for problems

Table 6.2 States with Mandatory Hospital Rate Regulation Programs

State	Inception Date
Colorado	1977
Connecticut	1974
Maryland	1973
Massachusetts	1971
New Jersey	1971
New York	1969
Rhode Island	1971
Washington	1973
Wisconsin	1975

Source: Department of Health, Education, and Welfare, American Hospital Association, and private communications.
Note: Inception dates vary by source reflecting in part changing statutory authorities.

HEW normally lists Rhode Island with the mandatory states even though the cooperative program between the state government, Blue Cross, and the hospital association is not mandated by statute. Hospitals must participate to get Blue Cross and Medicaid reimbursement, and coverage is 100 percent of hospitals. The AHA lists this as a voluntary program.

Table 6.3 States with Mandatory Advisory Hospital Rate Review Programs

State	Inception Date
Arizona	1972
Minnesota	1977
Oregon	1973
Virginia	1978

Source: American Hospital Association, private communications.

Table 6.4 States with Voluntary Private Rate Regulation Programs

State	Inception Date	Percentage of Hospitals Participating
Arkansas	1973	100
Delaware	1971	100
Florida	1976	88
Indiana	1959	100
Kansas	1976	83
Kentucky	1974	100
Michigan	1978	98
Missouri	1972	98
Montana	1971	82
New Hampshire	1976	52
Ohio	1948	19
Vermont	1976	100

Source: American Hospital Association.
Note: Nine of these programs are administered by Blue Cross, one by a hospital association, and two by joint commissions.

payers covered, resources devoted to regulatory efforts, and the extent of interaction and cooperation with providers and insurers. Table 6.5 lists some of the characteristics of the eight state regulatory programs that I have characterized as mandatory. Because this form of regulation is relatively new, because there were limited administrative models to follow, and because useful cost accounting and information collection systems did not exist, most of these agencies have continued to evolve. It is therefore useful to look more closely at the regulatory programs in several states.

New York
New York was the first state to adopt a mandatory reimbursement regulation program, and there is a general perception that this program places the greatest financial constraints on hospitals. Although the New York program is atypical in a number of ways, it is useful to examine it first because it has used so many of the reimbursement schemes.[28]

New York does not have a single independent regulatory commission with broad authority to set charges and reimbursement rates. State rate-setting depends on the activities of several state agencies. These activities are coordinated by the State Department

Table 6.5 Characteristics of Eight State Regulatory Programs

State	Regulatory Agency	General Methodology	Funding Source	Frequency of Review
Connecticut	Independent commission	Budget review, formula	State; federal grants	Annually and at time of change
Maryland	Independent commission	Budget review, negotiation, formula	State; federal grants	Annually and at time of change
Massachusetts	Independent commission	Budget review, formula	State; federal grants	At time of change
New Jersey	State department of health	Budget review, negotiation, formula	State; federal grants	Annually
New York	State executive branch offices.	Formula	State	Annually and at time of change
Rhode Island	State Government, hospital association, Blue Cross	Budget review, negotiation	NA	Annually
Washington	Independent commission	Budget review	State; hospitals; federal grants	Annually
Wisconsin	State hospital rate program	Budget review	Blue Cross; Medicaid program	At time of change

Source: American Hospital Association

of Health and are broadly administered by the Department's Division of Health Care Financing (DHCF) of the Office of Health Management Systems (OHMS). The commissioner of health must certify that the rates hospitals charge the state, private payers, and third-party payers are reasonable. For Medicaid rates this certification must be provided to the director of the budget; for Blue Cross rates, to the commissioner of insurance. Until 1978 only Medicaid and Blue Cross rates were subject to review by the Department of Health. In 1978 regulatory authority was extended to all hospital charges, including self-pay and privately insured patients. Hospitals are prohibited from raising daily charges except for adjustments approved by the state. Medicare rates were not covered by state regulation as of 1980.

To help determine reasonable costs and appropriate hospital charges, the DHCF has several bureaus. The Bureau of Hospital Rate Setting is responsible for determining the appropriate costs and cost relationships and for establishing rates for individual hospitals. This bureau is also responsible for receiving and deciding appeals. The Bureau of Economic Analysis calculates a trend factor based on a methodology established by an independent panel of health economists. This factor is used to make year-to-year adjustments in the base rates established by the Bureau of Hospital Rate Setting to reflect inflation and other trends that should be included in rate adjustments. The Bureau of Audits and Investigation collects and audits cost data from hospitals for use by the rate-setting bureaus.

Reimbursement rates for Medicaid and Blue Cross patients (accounting for about 50 percent of total hospital revenues) are based on a complicated set of formulas and trend factors. Hospitals are divided into comparable groups based on the number of beds, services offered, and teaching status. (The specific grouping method was changed in 1977.) Routine costs are arrayed according to cost per day, and ancillary costs according to costs per admission. Hospitals whose costs are (for example) above 125 percent or below 75 percent of the group mean are excluded, and a new group mean is calculated. Any hospital costs above the new group mean are excluded from reimbursement unless the hospital can win an appeal. The reimbursement formulas also include corrections or penalties for deviations from the group mean in average length of stay and target occupancy and utilization rates. The specific grouping criteria, adjustment methods, and penalty corrections have changed over time and differ between Medicaid and Blue Cross allowed per diem rates. The New York system penalizes hospitals that do not sustain target occupancy rates. For example, urban hospitals are expected to achieve medical-surgical occupancy rates of 85 percent, pediatric occupancy rates of 70 percent, and maternity unit occupancy rates of 60 percent. Hospitals that have lower occupancy rates have their actual patient-days adjusted to the level that would have yielded the required occupancy rate. This leads to a reduction in the per diem rate allowed, since the allowed per diem rate is (roughly) given by allowable costs divided by actual inpatient-days plus penalty inpatient-days.

These formulas are used to define base-level costs for each hospital, and trend factors reflecting inflation are used to adjust base costs to prospective reimbursement rates. These trend factors appear to underestimate the rate of change in input prices, and retroactive payments have had to be made. Furthermore, base-level costs have been adjusted very slowly.

The New York rate-setting system incorporates all three of the basic reimbursement regulation schemes discussed earlier in this chapter. A comparable-hospital approach is used to establish allowable costs for each hospital. A specific-criterion formula based on occupancy rate criteria is used to adjust allowed rates to a level below average cost for those hospitals that do not meet the criteria. Finally, by using an inflation adjustment factor that lags behind actual inflation and by updating base-level allowable costs slowly, the system indirectly gives many hospitals a binding general budget constraint. Whether this constraint is the intent of state regulatory authorities or merely the result of a time-consuming administrative system in a period of rapid inflation is unknown.[29]

The New York approach has placed severe financial pressure on hospitals in New York. As a group, New York community hospitals have sustained deficits during each of the years 1976 to 1978, and about 80 percent of New York hospitals had deficits in 1977 or 1978. The financial pressures have forced hospitals into backruptcy and have led to some consolidations. The hospitals have complained bitterly and have filed thousands of appeals and law suits. It could reasonably be argued, however, that if one wants to use financial constraints to reduce a perceived excess capacity and to constrain expansion, this is exactly what one has to expect, especially in the short run.

Massachusetts

In Massachusetts reimbursement regulation is the responsibility of the independent Rate Setting Commission (RSC) within the Executive Office of Human Services.[30] Although the Massachusetts Rate Setting Commission was established in 1968 and played a role in approving Medicaid reimbursement rates for hospitals during the early 1970s, the current structure is primarily the result of legislative changes made in 1973, 1975, and 1976. The RSC consists of three members appointed by the governor for three-year terms and has a staff of about 125. The state has also created a Hospital Policy Review Board to advise the RSC. This board has representatives from providers, insurers, and other government agencies concerned with hospital expenditures and the quality of care. As of 1980 the RSC had the following general responsibilities regarding hospitals:

To establish Medicaid reimbursement rates for each hospital.

To review and approve all hospital budgets, costs, and posted charges for individual services (affecting self-pay patients and patients with private insurance).

To review and approve contracts between Blue Cross and participating hospitals. The RSC does not have authority to specify the specific reimbursement contract but only to approve what is negotiated between Blue Cross and the hospitals.

Thus the RSC has direct control over about 30 percent of payments (Medicaid and charge based) and indirect control over all reimbursement excluding Medicare reimbursement. Until 1975 the RSC had direct control only over Medicaid reimbursements. Since 1976 the RSC has also regulated hospital charges and budgets as a result of changes in its legislative authority. Perhaps because of this historical dichotomy, two separate rate regulation systems have evolved—one for Medicaid reimbursement and one for charge control.

Let us consider the determination of Medicaid reimbursement rates first. The RSC determines a per diem rate for each hospital treating Medicaid patients. This rate is determined once a year and varies by hospital depending on a hospital's average costs per inpatient-day. Base-year costs are established for each hospital, using the costs incurred by the hospital two years before the year in which the rates are to be in effect. Operating costs are adjusted by a complex inflation index. Nonoperating costs (depreciation, interest) from the base year are then added without any inflationary adjustment. This gives the numerator of the formula for determining per diem reimbursement. These allowable costs are then divided by allowable inpatient-days to give the per diem Medicaid rate for each hospital. The inpatient-day figure is either actual inpatient-days during the base year or, if a hospital does not achieve minimum occupancy rates (65 percent for obstetric, 75 percent for pediatric, 80 percent for all other beds), a higher value is used to penalize the hospital for underutilization. This computation is similar to the New York penalty approach. The resulting rate then goes into effect for a year, subject to the requirement that it can be no higher than the Medicare cost limitation under section 223 of the Social Security Act Amendments of 1972 or the average charge per day for non-Medicaid patients. Outpatient expenditures are reimbursed based on average accounting costs for the base year unless these costs exceed the posted charges. Medicaid reimbursement does not allow for bad debts or free care, the costs of which must either be spread over other payers or absorbed by the hospital.

The charge control system, affecting patients insured with commercial insurers or uninsured patients, is considerably different from the methodology used to determine Medicaid reimbursements and has been changing over time. The RSC endeavors to establish a value of reasonable financial requirements for each hospital for the coming year and then establishes a set of routine and ancillary service charges that, given anticipated volumes, will yield net revenues equal to the hospital's financial requirements. This system yields a set of service charges rather than an all-inclusive per diem rate as used for Medicaid reimbursement.

To determine a hospital's reasonable financial requirements the RSC starts with the hospital's actual operating costs for a test year two years before the year the rates are to be in effect—the base-level costs. These costs are then adjusted by an inflation trend index developed by the RSC and approved projections made by the hospitals of volume changes from the base year through the rate year. Volume changes must increase by more than 3 percent or decrease by more than 5 percent to be included in the determination. Changes in operating costs associated with volume changes are calculated by assuming that the marginal cost is 40 percent of the base-year average cost. This gives the expected operating cost requirements for the rate year. Total financial requirements are then determined by adding items from the capital budget (interest, depreciation), a contribution for working capital, and certain approved cost increases outside the hospital's control. Allowed charges are then determined so that the expected revenue generated by these charges will equal the reasonable financial requirements of the hospital less expected payments from all cost-based third-party payers (Medicare, Medicaid, Blue Cross). Until 1980, the RSC paid relatively little attention to the precise relationship between individual posted charges and the related departmental average costs. However, the RSC is in the process of implementing a system that will eliminate any cross-subsidization resulting from the rate structure freedom previously given to hospitals.

There are a number of differences between the Massachusetts system and the New York system:

1. New York covers all patients except Medicare. Massachusetts covers only Medicaid, self-pay, and privately insured patients directly.

2. For rates in effect in 1979 and 1980 the Massachusetts RSC did not use a comparable-hospital approach or any similar approach to determine the reasonableness of the base-year costs reported by the hospitals (although this is being developed). New York has developed a complex grouping system to perform this type of analysis.

3. The Massachusetts RSC incorporates occupancy rate criteria only in its Medicaid reimbursement process. New York incorporates occupancy rate penalties in essentially all of the rates over which it has control.

4. Both states appear to have indirectly imposed somewhat more stringent budgetary constraints than the precise formulas might indicate by using fairly old historical data for establishing base-year costs and by using trend factors that have underestimated the general rate of inflation in input prices. The volume adjustment "corridors" used in Massachusetts add some additional constraint. The New York system appears to be more severe in this regard because it does not offer as much flexibility in projecting volume changes as does the Massachusetts RSC.

5. The Massachusetts RSC includes capital costs for projects approved by the CON authority without any lag on a pure cost pass-through basis. The combination of general formulas and

regulatory lag in New York limits this pass-through at least in terms of time.

In terms of the three generic reimbursement constraints, it appears that most of the power of the Massachusetts system comes from the interaction of limited volume adjustments, regulatory lag, and rapid inflation. The RSC has not historically used a comparable-hospital approach for determining reasonableness, uses a specific-criterion formula only for Medicaid reimbursement, has no general criterion for constraining increases in the volume of services, and does not cover even a majority of the payments to hospitals in Massachusetts. The system gets most of its "bite" by keeping reimbursement rates below inflationary increases in input prices, forcing hospitals to face real resource constraints to break even.

Washington

In 1973 the state of Washington created an independent regulatory commission to regulate hospital rates (the Washington State Hospital Commission, WSHC).[31] The commission has five members appointed by the governor for four-year terms. The commission must have at least one member representing consumers, labor, hospitals, and the business community. The rates established by the commission affect all payers, including Medicare, with a few exceptions.

The Washington system is a budget review and approval system that appears to involve considerable interaction and negotiation between the regulatory agency and the hospitals. The commission uses a variety of grouping and screening techniques to arrive at an approved budget for each hospital for the coming year. Rates are set for each department so that the total revenues expected to be generated by the departmental rates times the expected departmental volumes are equal to the approved budget. Although the WSHC was established in 1973, it took several years for it to develop an accounting and reporting system and a budget review and approval procedure. The first hospital budgets were not reviewed and approved until late 1976.

The budget approval system begins with submissions of budget information to the commission each year. Each hospital submits data on prior-year costs and utilization, current-year costs and utilization, and a projection for the next year's revenue requirements—the hospital's requested budget. Each hospital's projected operating expenses and its components are compared with the characteristics of one of the five peer groups into which each hospital is placed as well as with historical trends. If a particular hospital's projections are below the 70th percentile for its peer group for each of six screening variables, its operating expenses are approved. If a hospital's projections for each of six screening variables are above the 70th percentile, it is subjected to a more detailed screening process for a larger number of individual expense categories to determine why specific cost categories are above the 70th percentile. If, after this detailed analysis, the commission is not convinced that the differences are reasonable, it can recommend adjustments in hospital's allowed operating expenses. All projected hospital budgets are also subjected to general reviews of volume adjustments, capital expenditures, cross-subsidization between departments (no more than 5 percent), bad debts, and the like. The "reasonableness" criteria applied appear to be vague and subjective, and no significant constraints in these dimensions are evident.

This budget review process leads to a staff recommendation in the form of a total revenue requirement for the coming year and a set of departmental charges per unit of services. The staff also adjusts the actual reimbursement rates required from each major third-party payer to reflect historical reimbursement relationships, primarily in an effort to freeze the proportion of total revenue paid by each payer group to each hospital at levels prevailing before the creation of the new budget review and reimbursement system. For a variety of reasons Medicare and Blue Cross get a discount as a result of this process.

Since 1977, under a contract with the Social Security Administration, the WSHC has superimposed three separate experimental reimbursement systems on this budget review process. Hospitals are each placed in one of three reimbursement groups.

Group 1. Each participating third-party payer pays each hospital its fair proportion of the total budgeted revenue requirement as determined by the review process. Individuals and any third-party payers that are not part of the program pay the posted charges for services provided. Thus the hospitals in this group are basically assured that a large share of their budgeted revenues will be paid regardless of their actual cost and utilization experience.

Group 2. All payers pay the posted charges determined by the WSHC for each payer group (Blue Cross and Medicare get a credit) based on services provided.

Group 3. Conventional cost-based reimbursement is used by Medicare, Medicaid, and Blue Cross. Other payers pay the posted charges for service.

At the end of the year each hospital's experience is reviewed, and adjustments are made to account for revenue yields above or below budget. If a hospital reimbursed under group 1 receives less revenue than is budgeted, no automatic adjustments are made. If it receives more, part of the overrun is credited to the next year's budget. The adjustments are meant to reflect primarily differences between actual and projected service volumes.

Despite its computational complexity, the Washington State reimbursement system has many similarities to the traditional model of public utility regulation without significant regulatory lag. The system is primarily a process for reviewing projections of costs and volumes and assuring that reasonable cost and volume increases are fully reimbursed. The system contains no specific criterion-formula constraints based on occupancy rate or length of stay. The peer group analysis is used to identify outliers for further analysis, not as a formula for penalizing outliers in de-termining rates. Efforts are made to accommodate volume changes and intensity changes, not specifically to constrain them. Certain adjustments can be made retrospectively. Thus the Washington system is aimed primarily at ensuring that revenues will equal costs incurred. Thus we should not expect this type of system, with limited norms or constraints on the primary sources of re-source misallocation, to be very effective in containing hospital expenditures.

The remaining regulatory commissions follow procedures sim-ilar to one or more of these three states. The Connecticut, New Jersey, and Maryland processes now seem to lie, in terms of the imposition of real constraints on hospital behavior, somewhere between the extremes of New York and Washington. The general trend, however, also appears to be to adopt more of the normative criterion formulas used by New York but to apply more severe constraints gradually. Over time, most state rate-setting agencies have found it necessary to move beyond the naive public utility model, because its strict application is not a particularly potent constraint on hospital behavior. Efforts to develop criteria are still evolving, with New York having gone furthest toward a fairly rigid combination of the comparable-hospital and specific-criterion approaches combined with an implicit general budget constraint resulting from regulatory lag. In other states more informal general budget reviews based on projections of utilization, service changes, and inflationary factors are gradually being supplemented by more specific normative criteria based primarily on analyses of groups of comparable hospitals within the states. The ultimate outcome in these states depends heavily on a process of negotiation between the hospitals, the regulatory agency, and Blue Cross rather than on rigid formulas based on exogenous normative criteria. While the financial constraints imposed by other states do not appear to have been nearly as severe as those imposed in New York, they have not gone unchallenged in court.[32]

It is useful to present a simple generalization of the process that states go through or are moving toward in establishing prospective budgets or rates.

1. Establish base level costs (C) using the reasonableness criteria in effect in any particular state.

First, the regulatory authority examines the recent cost experience of a particular hospital for a base period, usually the most recent year. The starting point for determining the rate base would be the hospital's actual costs. However, costs may be disallowed or adjusted using comparable-hospital criteria or specific utilization criteria. This process may be applied to aggregate costs or to particular cost centers depending on the regulations in each state. Decisions must be made about the treatment of interest and depreciation. Adjustments for known changes, such as new facilities approved by CON agencies, may be incorporated.

2. Estimate expected changes in the prices of inputs over the period that rates will be in effect to find an inflation adjustment or trend factor (I).

3. Estimate expected changes in volume and the intensity of care that the hospital is likely to experience over the period that the rates are expected to be in effect to find a volume adjustment factor (V).

The prospective budget or service center rates approved would then be determined by the following formula:

$$B = C(1 + I)(1 + V).$$

The stringency of the regulatory constraint actually applied in any case depends on the ways in which these three factors are determined. In particular, the following considerations are of considerable importance:

1. A state commission could simply engage in an accounting exercise that yields a value for C that is whatever a particular hospital spent independent of any normative criteria. The use of comparable-hospital criteria introduces some additional constraint that should reduce organizational slack and perhaps encourage process innovation. The addition of specific utilization criteria to penalize underutilized facilities by adjusting the allowed rate base accordingly introduces an additional constraint that discourages facility duplication. As a result, this aspect of the budget or determination process varies from having no effect to constraining certain departures from cost-minimizing behavior.

2. In an inflationary world determining the inflation adjustment is of some significance. Underestimating input price changes and not allowing for retrospective recovery places an additional financial constraint on the hospital. Overestimating inflation and not allowing for retrospective recovery imposes no additional constraint over that implied by the determination of C and may actually reduce its stringency. Allowing for retrospective recovery for underestimates of input price changes eliminates the inflation adjustment factor as a constraint and may actually encourage increases in input prices, especially wages. Labor unions will probably favor adjustment factors that allow for retrospective recovery of wage increases.

3. The treatment of changes in the volume and intensity of care is important in determining whether a rate regulation program can really constrain the major source of increasing expenditures and inefficiency in the system. Regulatory systems that merely "pass through" volume and intensity increases by accepting hospital projections or making retrospective adjustments are simply reinforcing the primary dynamic forces leading to expenditure increases and inefficiency. Commissions that try to constrain volume or intensity increases through the use of normative criteria are likely to have the greatest long-run impact on hospital expenditures and performance. They will also run into the excess demand difficulties discussed before.

The evolution of rate regulation in most states seems to follow a similar pattern. Initial efforts are directed at developing reporting and accounting techniques that allow commissions to develop comparable base-line cost estimates for different hospitals. These are used in conjunction with simple estimates of inflation and historical changes in volume and intensity to establish an initial prospective budget criterion. Retrospective adjustments for errors in predicting inflation and volume increases are likely to be allowed. This is essentially an application of the naive public utility model and should have no more than a transitory effect on the system.

Rate-setting commissions later turn their attention to developing real normative criteria to help refine the value for C. Most commissions seem eventually to turn to a comparable-hospital approach. The commissions may also learn that the combination of inflation adjustment and regulatory lag puts additional pressure on the hospitals. In particular, they may allow retrospective recovery for unanticipated inflation only if the projection falls beyond some error band. At this stage commissions are still not likely to try to factor in normative criteria for utilization, volume, or intensity.

Eventually the commissions must decide whether they are going to put explicit constraints on utilization levels for particular types of facilities and for volume and intensity increases. State commissions are only now beginning to tackle the problems inherent in taking this step. New York has incorporated utilization criteria in the formula for determining C and has implicitly constrained V by freezing base-level costs at a specific level. Other state commissions seem to have embarked on this third step only very slowly and with great hesitation. However, this step has the greatest prospects for achieving long-term expenditure constraints of the magnitudes that the federal government seems to think are reasonable.

Other Government Constraints

The financial constraints placed on hospitals by state and federal authorities are probably more extensive than implied by a count of the states with mandatory rate review programs. Federal Medicare reimbursement policies and state Medicaid reimbursement and coverage provisions both have the potential for providing incentives to influence hospital supply decisions.

Efforts to cover the costs of hospitalization for the poor are concentrated primarily in state Medicaid programs. Criteria for eligibility, the extent of coverage, and reimbursement procedures vary enormously from state to state.[33] Although the federal government reimburses the state for 50 to 70 percent of the costs of the Medicaid programs, state differences in eligibility, coverage, income distribution, and hospital costs have led to large differences in the burden that Medicaid costs put on state budgets. As hospital costs have grown, states with relatively generous benefit plans and large welfare populations have found it more and more difficult to finance Medicaid programs. A number of states have cut back Medicaid benefits and adjusted reimbursement formulas to reduce the relative payments that hospitals receive for serving Medicaid patients. In states like New York and Massachusetts, it has been argued that cutbacks on coverage and reimbursement rates have placed severe financial constraints on a large number of hospitals.[34] In short, state efforts to reduce Medicaid expenditures have placed increasing general budgetary pressures on hospitals, and they must respond either by reducing expenditures or by going out of business. Although the intent of state efforts to reduce Medicaid expenditures is to help balance the state budget, the imposition of fiscal constraints on hospitals means that such efforts can become significant "indirect" instruments for constraining hospital supply behavior.

Finally, the federal government's Medicare reimbursement procedures may also place indirect constraints on hospital expenditures. Current reimbursement procedures discourage cross-subsidization, put some reasonableness constraints on routine care costs, provide lower contributions for depreciation than they once did (and some have argued inadequate depreciation allowances),[35] and will not cover any bad debts for non-Medicare patients. The larger a state's Medicare population, the more important are the effects of these reimbursement policies on the hospital's freedom to expand services and cover the costs of providing care.

In summary, experience with state regulation of hospital charges, budgets, and reimbursement rates is fairly limited. State programs have generally evolved from concern about the increasing burden on state budgets of public assistance programs and increases in Blue Cross premiums. The coverage of these programs has been expanding, but there is considerable diversity among the states in organizational structure, regulatory procedures, and formulas used for establishing reimbursement allowances. The diversity of the programs and the relatively short period that many have been operating make broad generalizations difficult. Formal state control of hospital reimbursement is concentrated primarily in the Northeast. In many states Blue Cross plans appear to prefer to use their power over hospital reimbursement to develop private restrictions on hospital reimbursement through negotiation rather than by state fiat. There is no evidence that the rate of diffusion of state reimbursement regulation will increase or soon attain the pervasive status of certificate-of-need regulation. States without general reimbursement regulation programs may still exert some financial constraints on hospital behavior through their control of Medicaid reimbursement rates and eligibility for benefits. Formal federal controls have been limited to certain reimbursement ceiling and accounting cost conventions used in determining Medicare reimbursement. Since the Medicare consumption of hospital services is fairly large (30 percent on average), these reimbursement rules may also place some financial constraint on hospitals with relatively large Medicare patient loads.

The Carter Administration's Cost Containment Proposals

The lack of a comprehensive federal reimbursement regulation program is not the result of disinterest on the part of federal authorities or the result of a failure to try to implement a national program. Because of the escalating financial burdens of the Medicare and Medicaid programs, the Carter administration was keenly interested in establishing a national program to control hospital expenditures. During his administration, President Carter proposed two similar national cost containment programs.

Program 1

In April 1977, soon after taking office, the Carter administration proposed the Hospital Cost Containment Act of 1977 (HR 6575 and S 1391).[36] The proposed program had two primary components. First, the act called for setting a ceiling on the revenues that any acute hospital could collect in any year from all payers. Second, the act provided for a national ceiling on approvals of new capital expenditures by acute hospitals.

The Revenue Ceiling   The act specified a formula for determining a national value for percentage increases in total inpatient revenues from one year to the next. The allowed percentage increase in revenues, applicable to virtually all acute hospitals in the country would have been calculated as the sum of the GNP deflator for the most recent 12-month period plus one-third of the difference between the average annual rate of increase in hospital expenditures in the preceding two years and the increase in the GNP deflator in the same period. Thus the ceiling provided for increases in revenues equal to a measure of general inflation in the economy plus a small declining allowance for real increases in expenditure. The structure of the formula for determining the basic limit meant that the allowed real increase in expenditures (assuming that the GNP deflator appropriately reflected changes in hospital input prices) would asymptotically approach zero with a large reduction from the historical trend in the first year of the program. The basic limit effectively provided for a very severe constraint on real expenditure growth.

The act also provided for certain adjustments to the basic limit. For increases in admission of more than 2 percent over the base-period level, a hospital could add 50 percent of the base-year revenue per stay to the ceiling for each admission beyond 2 percent of the base. If admissions declined more than 6 percent from the base-period level, a reduction of the ceiling equal to 50 percent of the revenue per stay would be applied for each admission below the 6 percent corridor. Hospitals would also have been allowed to adjust the revenue ceiling to reflect fully increases in wages to nonsupervisory personnel.

An administrative procedure to account for exceptional changes in patient load or major changes in capacity or services was also provided. To receive any additional revenue allowance, however, the hospital would also have had to show that without it, its financial performance would have fallen in the bottom quartile for all hospitals in the country.

In summary, the proposed cost containment system would have worked as follows. Each hospital would have started with its expenditures for the previous year, multiplied them by one plus the national allowable growth factor determined by the formula, and added adjustments for any wage increases and volume increases allowed. This figure would be its allowed budget for the year. The ceiling revenues allowed would then be applied to payments from all payers. Hospitals operating in states that had approved state reimbursement regulation programs and agreed to comply with the federal ceilings would be exempt from the federal cost containment program. Since a state program had to adhere to the federal guidelines to receive approval, this exemption was of little practical importance.

The proposed plan had several drawbacks. First, since the formula applied to increases in revenues from base-year levels and did not distinguish among hospitals with regard to the base level of expenditures, all hospitals in the country faced the same sharp constraint on real expenditure growth regardless of their current sophistication or level of efficiency. No distinction was made between costly sophisticated hospitals and less costly hospitals with limited service availabilities as of the base year. Second, the inflation adjustment was to be based on the GNP deflator for the entire country rather than on actual input price changes affecting individual hospitals. Third, the formula allowed only very limited increases in real expenditure growth except those provided for by the volume adjustments. Volume increases would have effectively been reimbursed at only 50 percent of historical cost regardless of the nature of the increased load or its costs.

The proposed revenue limits are an example of the general budget constraint instrument discussed before. The proposed Carter program had all the theoretical strengths and weaknesses of that instrument when implemented in a way that imposed a severe real resource constraint on hospitals.

Capital Expenditure Constraints   In addition to the ceilings on allowed hospital revenues, the act also provided for a national ceiling on new capital expenditures by hospitals. The proposal would have limited new capital expenditures by hospitals to $2.5 billion per year. (In 1978 capital expenditures by hospitals amounted to over $8 billion.) The national capital expenditure ceiling was to be allocated to the individual states by a formula, in the first instance according to state populations. The ceiling was to be applied by state CON agencies or by the federal government in states without CON agencies. The act also included maximum bed/population criteria and minimum occupancy rate criteria. Areas that did not satisfy these guidelines could not receive a certificate-of-need for new facilities that would have led to a net increase in beds.

It is not clear why the administration felt compelled to add the capital expenditure restrictions to the bill. The revenue restrictions should have been sufficient to accomplish almost any cost containment goal efficiently. As a result, the capital expenditure constraint seems to have been redundant. It may have been included for several reasons. First, the federal cost containment efforts had become wedded to the planning-CON model. Merely using a general budget constraint would naturally have led to questions about the need for the huge planning-CON bureaucracy that had been created. The entrenched planning bureaucracy within HEW certainly would not have been happy about that. Second, the administration may have become concerned that if the CON process proceeded without a capital constraint, continued approvals of most "needed" capital projects would have formed the basis for exceptions procedures under the act. Third, the authors of the legislation may simply have failed to think through the nature of the constraints that were to be applied and did not recognize that the capital constraint was redundant.

The Congressional Budget Office (CBO) estimated that if the act had been passed and worked as planned, it would have yielded hospital expenditures over a five-year period of $46 billion less than was expected without any federal constraints.[37] This would have been accomplished by limiting real expenditure growth to about 25 percent of what would otherwise have been expected. The CBO also identified a number of problems with the bill, including the arbitrary values used for the limits, the equal treatment of unequal hospitals, and the consequences of a sudden reduction in the real dynamic growth of the system on patients.

The administration's stringent constraint attracted considerable opposition to the proposal. It was opposed by the American Hospital Association, the Federation of American Hospitals, the American Medical Association, the Business Roundtable, representatives of rural areas and southern states, the National Association of Manufacturers, and many others.[38] Representative David Stockman prepared a very detailed and sophisticated attack on the proposed program and its underlying rational.[39] Health insurers supported the bill, but with many reservations. Both opponents and proponents agreed with the administration's broad objectives, but there was little enthusiastic support for the detailed proposal itself.

Program 2
In March 1979 the Carter administration submitted a second cost containment proposal, The Hospital Cost Containment Act of 1979.[40] This proposal followed the creation of a voluntary effort

to contain costs by the American Hospital Association, the Federation of American Hospitals, and the American Medical Association in late 1977. In an effort to head off mandatory federal and state regulation, these provider groups promoted voluntary arrangements, based on voluntary cost containment goals and cooperation between hospitals, third party-payers, and state agencies. The AHA claimed that the voluntary efforts were working, and it is in this context that the second cost containment program was introduced to Congress.

The revised cost containment proposals had many similarities to the original proposals. Changes reflected the need to respond to the voluntary efforts that were being advertised (and which the administration correctly believed could not work in the long run), the political fate of the first proposals, and the need for several technical refinements in the original proposals. The proposed legislation established a *national voluntary limit* on expenditure increases for hospitals for the next year (1979). If the hospital industry failed to meet the national voluntary limit, *standby mandatory controls* would have been applied to individual hospitals beginning in 1980. The national voluntary limit on increased expenditures was to be set as the sum of a market basket inflation index reflecting the costs of hospital inputs, 0.8 percent for population growth, and 1.0 percent for real increases in service intensity. HEW originally estimated that the ceiling would be 9.7 percent. In reality the ceiling would have been greater than 11 percent since inflation was greater than anticipated. Actual expenditure growth was over 13 percent, so the hospital industry would not have met the voluntary limits; and had the bill been passed the mandatory limits would have been activated.[41]

Under the mandatory program each hospital was to be given a ceiling on allowed increases in expenditures. The basic limit was to be set equal to the individual hospital's "market basket" price increases. To this would be added a bonus for efficiency or a penalty for inefficiency. Whether hospitals were efficient or inefficient would have been determined by comparing their routine costs per day with the median and variance of these costs for groups of comparable hospitals. No adjustments were to be made for hospitals that fell within 115 percent of the group median. Those above 115 percent of the group median would have received a penalty, those below would have received a bonus. The bonuses and penalties ranged from $+1.0$ percent to -2.0 percent. Additional adjustments were to be allowed for changes in the volume of care. An exceptions procedure was also included.

The act also included more exemptions than the previous one. If a state achieved the voluntary limit in the aggregate in 1979, all hospitals in the state would be exempt from mandatory controls in 1980. Hospitals in states with approved state cost containment programs would have been exempt. Very small hospitals and HMO hospitals would also have been exempt.

The second cost containment program was different from the first in a number of ways. In effect, the program ceded more responsibility to the states, since all hospitals in a state could avoid federal regulation if the state could meet the voluntary limits in the aggregate. Second, rather than the GNP deflator, actual hospital input price indexes would be used. Third, efforts would be made to differentiate between efficient and inefficient hospitals using some kind of comparable hospital formula. The act did not include a capital expenditure ceiling, although one was included in the administration's national health insurance proposals (which Congress did not pass). However, the bottom line was the same. Federal regulation would be triggered if the hospital sector could not reduce the real rate of growth in expenditures by perhaps 70 percent. The mandatory limits imposed what may have turned out to be even more restrictive budget constraints than the original proposals. The 1979 bill was opposed by essentially the same groups that opposed the first set, and the act was not passed by Congress.

The Carter administration therefore tried to impose general budget constraints on hospitals. The general approach had considerable merit. Unfortunately, the administration tried to do too much too soon and oversold the program. Whether they believed it or not, administration representatives continually argued that the cost containment objectives could be achieved easily by eliminating waste and inefficiency of no benefit to patients. Indeed, HEW Secretary Califano's estimates of the savings to be achieved by eliminating excess beds increased by a factor of more than two between 1977 and 1979.[42] There is little reason to believe that there is so much slack in the system. Financial constraints of this magnitude would reduce the benefits of hospital care that would otherwise be available, perhaps in inequitable ways. By recognizing that some sacrifices must be made (at least dynamically), a regulatory program such as the one proposed would at least have been better able to deal with the allocative and distribution issues that naturally arise. Whether admitting the truth makes the political prospects of implementing this type of legislation more attractive is another question. Resolving this conflict between reducing expenditures and reducing benefits will be a critical element of any public policy aimed at improving resource allocation in this sector, whether they be regulatory instruments or some nonregulatory alternative.

Conclusions

It does not appear that any form of administrative regulation offers an easy or comprehensive solution to the problems that motivated our interest in public interventions. This does not mean, however, that some forms of government regulation of hospitals are not preferable to others or that the best of the imperfect regulatory schemes do not lead to resource allocation superior to the status quo. Just because we cannot expect regulatory interventions to solve all the problems does not mean that they cannot help solve some of them.

CON regulation will almost always be dominated by some form of reimbursement regulation. A reimbursement constraint system can do essentially everything a CON system can do, and it can do it more quickly and efficiently. Furthermore, it promotes additional efficiencies that CON does not.

Some form of general budget constraint or the combination of a general budget constraint with comparable-hospital and specific-criterion reimbursement formulas has many attractive properties and appears to be the most desirable of the alternative regulatory instruments. It runs into two problems. If it does not attempt to account for significant differences between hospitals and their patient populations, it can lead to undesirable allocative outcomes and run into severe political difficulties. In addition, if the constraint applied is too severe, the induced excess demand and associated nonprice rationing of demand raises difficult efficiency, equity, and political problems. It appears, then, that if a regulatory strategy is to be adopted, it makes sense to start with the development of comparable-hospital and specific-criterion formulas and gradually to superimpose increasingly severe general budget constraints. This allows inefficiencies associated with non-cost-minimizing behavior to be squeezed out first. Then the care with extremely low values relative to costs could be rationed, and the constraints could be gradually tightened as far as the political system will allow. Exactly how far we can go is an empirical question. We can squeeze something from the system by following this strategy, but probably not nearly as much as most policymakers would like.

This tentative regulatory strategy leaves no room for CON regulation. A question that naturally arises is whether we should have CON regulation as well. The answer is probably no. We certainly do not want to encourage the development of separate CON and reimbursement regulatory systems. This would lead to either redundant regulations or undesirable conflicts between regulatory agencies. Conflicts are of special concern here if we believe that the most potent of the regulatory instruments is some form of incentive-oriented reimbursement constraints. If CON agencies are allowed to operate separate from reimbursement agencies, any facility that gets a certificate of need will almost certainly have a legal claim to reimbursement. If CON agency objectives conflict with those of reimbursement agencies, a CON agency could easily restrict the ability of the reimbursement authority to develop criteria for improving resource allocation. At the very least, CON processes should be integrated fully with reimbursement constraint policies. There are good practical as well as theoretical reasons to scrap the CON process almost entirely and to stop relying on it to make a significant contribution to improvements in resource allocation and reductions in hospital expenditures.

The Effects of Government Regulation

Since many states have had several years of experience with certificate-of-need or reimbursement regulation, we would expect to be able to observe some effects if these regulatory schemes have been effective. If we cannot observe significant effects, this does not necessarily mean that they cannot have effects on facility expansion, hospital utilization, and total hospital expenditures, but only that any anticipated effects must be based on theoretical considerations rather than historical evidence.

The discussion in chapters 5 and 6 led to a number of tentative hypotheses. First, CON regulation is most likely to reflect the weak considerations inherent in the first model of CON agency objectives rather than the strong considerations involving binding capacity constraints inherent in CON2. Second, most CON behavior has focused on acute hospital bed supplies and only to a lesser extent on ancillary facilities. Third, for these reasons and a variety of other restrictions on the extent of CON regulation, I would expect to find some evidence that bed supplies have been affected but that the effects on total hospital expenditures will be small. Fourth, regulation of hospital reimbursement has the prospect of achieving much larger responses by the hospital sector, but these regulations are likely to be most effective where formal or implicit normative criteria for reviewing hospital budgets and hospital reimbursement rates have been translated into binding budgetary constraints. Fifth, hospitals in states with generous Medicaid programs and states with large Medicare populations are most likely to be affected by increasingly restrictive reimbursement policies.

It is unreasonable to expect instantaneous effects of any of these regulatory programs. Regulatory agencies often take many years to become mature in terms of their analytical capabilities to affect hospital behavior and the fraction of hospital facilities and expenditures that can be controlled by either statute or regulation. We should probably not be surprised to find that significant effects of these regulations do not appear until the mid 1970s. By then many states had several years of experience with these regulatory instruments. In addition, this was the period in which federal interest in cost containment increased substantially and state fiscal problems began to be at least partially identified with escalating Medicaid costs. Also, we are likely to observe the effects of binding reimbursement constraints much more quickly than capital expenditure constraints.

Previous Empirical Studies

Several studies of the effects of certificate-of-need regulation and reimbursement regulation have appeared in the literature, all based primarily on data prior to 1975. In a much cited study Salkever and Bice examined state data on changes in total plant assets, total beds, plant assets per bed, and per capita hospital costs for the period 1968–1972 to determine the effects of certificate-of-need regulation.[1] CON regulation was measured either by a dummy variable that was equal to unity if a state had a CON program in effect for at least two quarters in any year and zero otherwise, or by a variable equal to the fraction of the 1968–1972 period that a CON program was in place. They found that CON regulation reduced the growth rate in beds but increased the growth rate in assets per bed. Salkever and Bice interpret this result as implying that CON's constraint on bed supplies induced a substitution of other forms of capital investment for bed investments. They also found that states with CON programs had slightly higher growth rates in costs per capita.

While these results are not theoretically implausible, I feel that the CON programs in this study were in place for too short a period to have had any significant effects and that the perverse effects associated with the CON variable are probably due to other factors. In particular, it is not unreasonable to assume that CON regulations were first introduced in states with higher than average per capita hospital costs and perhaps in response to rapid growth in sophisticated ancillary services. I find Salkever and Bice's arguments about preemptive investment completely implausible. Relatively long lead times are needed to observe changes in investment plans in capital stocks, and it is a reasonable assumption that CON regulations would take several years to become a serious constraint on hospital behavior.

Hellinger used cross-sectional state data for the period 1971–1973 to examine the effects of CON regulation on total plant assets and total investment.[2] In his examination of total assets for 1973, CON regulation is measured by a dummy variable equal to unity if a state had a program in effect on January 1 of that year. His analysis of total plant assets for 1971 and 1972 used a CON dummy variable indicating whether a CON law was passed during the first nine months of that year. (This is really an investment equation for 1971 and 1972 because total plant assets lagged one year appear as an independent variable.) Hellinger found that CON regulation had an insignificant effect on total plant assets in 1973 and that the passage of CON regulation in 1971 and 1972 had a significant positive effect on the rate of investment in those years. He interprets the second set of results as implying the existence of preemptive investments. For exactly the same reasons that I question the robustness of Salkever and Bice's results, I feel that Hellinger's results must also be taken with a grain of salt.

Sloan and Steinwald use cross-sectional data on a large sample of community hospitals to examine the effects of a wide range of regulatory variables on hospital costs and input use for the period 1970 to 1975.[3] Five variables designed to capture differences in CON programs are utilized, two variables to measure the presence of section 1122 agreements and Blue Cross approval requirements are included, and two variables are used to indicate the existence of some form of prospective reimbursement program. The overall results indicate that regulatory variables have either insignificant or positive (perverse) effects on hospital costs. There is some evidence that budget-based prospective reimbursement programs reduced hospital costs and that Blue Cross approval requirements did so as well. The magnitudes of these effects are small. On the input side, the results appear to indicate that CON regulations have stimulated bed growth and had an insignificant effect on assets per bed. Overall, they conclude that during this period state regulatory variables showed little constraining effect on hospital costs.

In a more recent paper I examined the effects of hospital regulation and interhospital competition on hospital bed supply decisions in the context of a simple queuing model that focuses on the reservation quality of hospitals given a stochastic demand for services.[4] A sample of 346 private nonprofit hospitals in 1976 is used for the empirical work. I found that CON regulation and prospective reimbursement programs have consistently negative (constraining) effects on hospital reserve margins and associated bed supplies. The effects of CON regulation are not significantly different from zero when a simple dummy variable indicating the presence or absence of such programs is used. When the number of years that a program has been in effect is used (linearly and nonlinearly) however, the effect of CON regulation on hospital reserve margins is negative and quite significant. I attribute this result both to agency learning and to the fact that CON regulation, since it directly affects only the flow of beds, has significant effects on bed stocks only over a period of years. The results for the prospective reimbursement variable are less precise but uniformly negative.

A report prepared by Policy Analysis, Inc., done under contract with the Department of Health, Education, and Welfare, provides perhaps the most comprehensive descriptive and statistical analyses of CON programs and their effects on the level and rate of change in hospital costs.[5] This study makes a concerted effort to develop and discuss the differences between state CON programs and to develop numerical indexes reflecting the strictness of CON programs in different states. The empirical work is based largely on the data used by Sloan and Steinwald, augmented in a variety of ways and extended to cover 1976. The study finds that CON programs alone have little independent effect on the level or rate of growth in hospital costs, but direct rate regulation appears to have a significant effect on the rate of growth in hospital expenditures. This study also presents some evidence that the earliest states to institute CON programs tended to have much higher costs per day or per admission before the establishment of regulatory authority than did other states. The report quite correctly does not try to attribute this to preemptive behavior.

The evidence based on pre-1976 data seems to be that CON regulation may have had some effect on the supply of hospital beds but little apparent effect on total hospital expenditures. Some papers have concluded that the higher costs or higher investment levels observed in states that first instituted CON programs reflect perverse responses. I think it is more likely, given the time frame in which these analyses were done, that the causality goes the other way. There is also some evidence that reimbursement regulation and active Blue Cross constraint programs have dampened the growth in hospital expenditures.[6] At least up to 1976, however, the overall effects of economic regulation on hospital behavior and performance are not impressive.

Further Empirical Analysis

I turn now to an effort to supplement these earlier studies with some additional analysis using data covering the period through 1979. The three to five years of experience beyond that of previous studies allows us to focus on a much longer period of extensive regulatory activity. I propose to present some simple statistical analyses to explore whether recent experience provides additional information about the nature and size of the effects of the regulatory programs discussed here. It is essential to analyze more recent data because only in the last few years have state regulatory agencies begun to take their cost control mandates seriously and had the authority and capacity to implement cost containment objectives. I attack the problem in four related ways. First, I compare behavior between Pennsylvania and New York before and after 1975. These states are comparable except that Pennsylvania has imposed few regulatory constraints while New York has imposed nearly all of them. The year 1975 is chosen as the break point to differentiate between the phasing-in of regulation in New York and the ultimate effects of regulatory efforts that must be observed with some lag. I then examine aggregate experience on costs for all states with mature state reimbursement regulation programs and mature certificate-of-need programs in comparison with states lacking such programs. Third, I present a more comprehensive statistical analysis of the effects of CON regulation and state reimbursement regulation programs on the growth rate in hospital costs over the period 1973–1979. Finally, I examine the diffusion of CT scanners among the states to see whether facility regulation or reimbursement regulation has had constraining effects on a specific ancillary service that has attracted enormous attention.

New York's extensive cost containment, rate regulation, and certificate-of-need programs are generally acknowledged to be the most intensive regulatory programs in the country.[7] These government programs have been supplemented by independent efforts by Blue Cross to contain costs. The combination of enormous Medicaid expenditures plus serious state budget problems has forced New York to cut back on Medicaid reimbursements and to impose long repayment lags. There exists a large uncovered population, and bad debts have been growing. New York also has one of the oldest and largest prepaid group health plans in the country, providing some competition for the fee-for-service sector.[8] If regulation has been effective anywhere, New York is the most likely place.

Pennsylvania does not have a comprehensive state cost and rate regulation program, did not have a state certificate-of-need program until 1979, has not experienced New York's fiscal problems, and does not appear to have made cuts in Medicaid reimbursements of the same order of magnitude. The state has less than 10 percent of the enrollment in prepaid group plans than does New York.[9] A prospective reimbursement plan has been operated by Blue Cross in Western Pennsylvania, however. Both New York and Pennsylvania are large northeastern industrial states and have experienced essentially no population growth during the past decade.

Table 7.1 presents data on hospital expenditures and utilization for New York and for Pennsylvania. I have divided the data into two periods: preconstraint period (1971–1975) and a constraint period (1975–1979), reflecting hypothesized regulatory constraints imposed in New York but not in Pennsylvania.

The information presented in the table indicates that there have been some major changes in the trends of expenditures and uti-

Table 7.1 Hospital Expenditures and Hospital Utilization, Community Hospitals (compound rates of growth)

	New York		Pennsylvania	
	1971–1975	1975–1979	1971–1975	1975–1979
Expenditures	13.7	8.2	12.7	15.1
Hospitals	−1.7	−2.7	−0.2	0.5
Beds	0.5	−1.3	0.4	0.6
Admissions	0.9	−0.4	1.6	1.3
Adjusted Patient-Days	1.4	−0.4	0	1.1
Average Cost per Stay	12.4	8.2	10.0	13.0
Average Cost per Stay (dollars)				
1971	$1,135		$ 796	
1979	$2,228		$1,723	

lization in New York, in sharp contrast with the experience in Pennsylvania. During the 1971–1975 period hospital expenditures, adjusted patient-days, and the average cost per stay grew faster in New York than in Pennsylvania. The number of beds grew at about the same rate, although the number of hospitals declined at a much faster rate in New York, perhaps reflecting the fact that New York has had a certificate-of-need program since the mid 1960s, the first in the country.[10] In the 1975–1979 period the absolute and relative patterns for New York changed dramatically. Total expenditures grew at a rate less than half of Pennsylvania's and just about half of the national average rate. The rate of decline in the number of hospitals in New York accelerated, and beds, admissions, and adjusted patient-days all declined in New York while they continued to increase in Pennsylvania. The average cost per stay in New York in the latter period just about kept up with changes in input prices. Increases in the average cost per stay in Pennsylvania were about 5 percentage points above the rate of growth in input prices. Note, however, that in 1971 New York had a substantially higher cost per stay than Pennsylvania and that despite the constraints on expenditure and utilization growth, the cost per stay remains higher in New York than in Pennsylvania.

New York may be a polar example since hospitals in no other state have been forced to deal with such severe budgetary constraints. It is fairly clear, however, that tightening the budgetary constraints forces hospitals to respond. In New York they have responded by going out of business, merging, reducing the number of admissions, reducing some outpatient services, and constraining the real rate of growth in expenditures per case. Although New York started off with much more resource intensive and costly hospital care than Pennsylvania and has remained a higher-cost state, these effects have not been achieved without controversy.[11] Furthermore, there is some indication that the individuals who have been the most affected by these cutbacks are those with the poorest access to high-quality medical care.[12] Whether these constraints have affected health outcomes we do not yet know.

Comparing New York's experience with that of a comparable state and with the rest of the country indeed implies that the financial constraints imposed by state reimbursement policy and perhaps independent capital expansion constraints have reduced the growth rate in expenditures, utilization, and facilities.[13] Whether these kinds of constraints can be sustained in the face of opposition by providers, community groups, and patients only time will tell.[14] Presumably, it was easier to cut the growth rate in expenditures in New York than it might have been in a state that started out with less intensive and costly hospital care. However, the effect of regulation in New York may be diminishing. The reductions in admissions and inpatient-days in New York occurred primarily before 1979. In 1979 admissions and inpatient-days in New York increased at the same or higher rates than in Pennsylvania, and the difference in the rates of expenditure growth has narrowed considerably. Even New York may be running into diminishing returns in "squeezing" the system, as the resource constraints become harder and harder to accommodate without serious dislocations.

Given the apparent success of regulation in New York, I next ask whether other states with formal programs to regulate hospital reimbursement rates and facility expansion have been willing and able to squeeze the system as much as New York has. Table 7.2 presents data on recent expenditure experience among the states, classified by type of regulation. It is immediately apparent that the states with mandatory regulation of hospital budgets or charges as a group experienced a significantly lower rate of growth in total expenditures and expenditures per patient-day[15] than did the rest of the states in the country over the 1975–1979 period. This is true even if New York is excluded. This group of states also had a significantly lower growth rate in expenditures during the 1973–1975 period, however, even though several of these states had not yet established comprehensive reimbursement reg- ulation procedures during this period. During both time periods every state in the group experienced lower expenditure growth than the mean for the rest of the states in the population. But on the average the differences are much greater during the 1975–1979 period than during the 1973–1975 period.

Public discussions extolling the effects of state reimbursement regulation do not appear to have noted that the states with rate regulation programs generally tend to have been high-cost states at the time regulatory enforcement began in earnest. Consider first the data reported for cost per admission in table 7.2. Seven of the eight states with rate regulatory programs have higher costs per stay than the rest of the population in both 1975 and 1979.

Table 7.2 Comparisons between Regulated and Unregulated States

States	Change in Total Expenses (%)		Change in Cost per Day (%)		Cost per Admission ($)		Personnel per Bed	
	1975–1979	1973–1975	1975–1979	1973–1975	1975	1979	1975	1979
A. States with Mandatory Rate Regulatory Programs								
Connecticut	57.4	28.6	49.8	24.9	1,233	1,835	3.00	3.32
Maryland	68.9	33.4	51.5	27.3	1,277	1,946	3.02	3.22
Massachusetts	51.7	34.3	48.9	30.6	1,495	2,286	3.31	3.55
New Jersey	57.0	38.3	52.5	27.2	1,100	1,668	2.44	2.66
New York	37.0	33.7	39.8	28.1	1,628	2,230	3.02	3.17
Rhode Island	51.0	35.5	48.1	35.5	1,288	1,916	3.41	3.77
Washington	70.0	35.0	59.4	29.8	844	1,360	2.56	2.94
Wisconsin	69.5	31.8	69.0	27.4	939	1,573	2.20	2.54
Simple Means for Eight-State Group	57.8	33.8	52.3	28.9	1,225	1,819	2.87	3.14
B. Simple Means for Remaining States	80.6	38.3	70.0	31.5	867	1,464	2.39	2.65
C. Simple Means for States with CON Programs Prior to 1975	73.9	37.3	64.0	30.9	1,003	1,611	2.54	2.81
D. Same as C Excluding States in A	80.5	38.5	69.2	31.6	906	1,509	2.39	2.66
E. Means for States without CON Prior to 1975	80.3	37.9	70.0	31.3	840	1,434	2.38	2.64

Source: Based on data from Hospital Statistics, various years.

The same general pattern is observed in 1971 as well. On average the difference is about 50 percent in 1975 and 30 percent in 1978. New York and Massachusetts have substantially larger differences. Although the difference in cost per stay between the regulated and the unregulated states has declined (proportionally), the regulated states continue to exhibit higher costs per admission on average. These differences cannot be explained by adjusting for state-to-state differences in wages.

Similar patterns are observed when we look at the data on personnel per bed. We can assume that states with a greater number of employees per bed have either more intensive and technologically sophisticated hospital care, that they are supplying hospital care inefficiently, or some combination of both. On average states with reimbursement regulation had 20 percent more personnel per bed in 1975 than did the rest of the population, and this proportional difference declined only slightly by 1979. In both 1975 and 1979 seven of the eight regulated states had a ratio of personnel to beds above the mean for the rest of the states, and in some cases the difference is as much as 40 percent.

Finally, if we focus on Washington and Wisconsin, whose costs per admission and personnel per bed were closest to the mean for the unregulated states in 1975, we also find the smallest apparent effects of regulation on expenditure growth and unit costs. Regulation appears to have been most constraining in those states that had the highest costs per admission and historically provided the most intensive care to patients.

This simple data manipulation exercise leads to a number of tentative conclusions about the regulated states and helps to explain some of the results reported in previous econometric work. First, the states that initiated rate regulation earliest were those that had high costs per stay and had hospitals offering the most sophisticated hospital care. It should not be surprising that regression equations relating unit costs to input and regulatory variables reveal that states with rate regulation tend to have higher costs than those without it. Rather than represent a perverse effect of regulation, this result almost certainly reflects the fact that the high-cost states had the most interest in regulating hospital budgets and charges. Second, states that have established comprehensive reimbursement regulation programs have tended to experience a slower rate of growth in expenditures and unit costs than the rest of the population, especially the six high-cost states in the group. This may be attributable entirely to regulatory initiatives, or it could be partly the result of natural dynamic cycles in technological change, where the high costs in these states represent an early exploitation of available quality opportunities and where the rest of the states have been catching up.[16] To get some feeling for whether this is merely a spurious relationship, reflecting a general tendency of the higher-cost, more sophisticated hospital systems to be experiencing less rapid expenditure growth, it is useful to look at high-cost states that are not regulated. Table 7.3 presents expenditure data for the next six high-cost states (including Washington, D.C.) that do not have reimbursement regulation. While these states have somewhat lower growth in total expenditures in the 1975–1979 period than the rest of the unregulated states, the changes in cost per day and cost per admission are just about the same. The eight regulated states as a group have a significantly lower rate of growth in expenditures per day than the unregulated states whether they have high or low base-level costs. Any differences between the unregulated states, in terms of expenditure growth, is probably attributable largely to differences in population growth. The data therefore continue to be consistent with the hypothesis that reimbursement regulation has constrained the growth rate in unit expenditures.

When we sort states according to the presence or absence of CON regulation prior to 1975, we find essentially no evidence that CON regulation alone has any significant effect on expenditure and unit cost growth or that there are particularly large differences in cost per admission or personnel per bed. (Compare D and E in table 7.2.) To the extent that there are any apparent effects of CON regulation on any of these variables, it appears to be due entirely to the simultaneous existence of state rate regulation programs. (Compare C and D.) The Policy Analysis study, using sophisticated econometric techniques, came to essentially the same conclusion. States that initiated only CON programs before 1975 tend to have slightly higher costs per admission in 1979 than the unregulated states, but the differences are not statistically significant. In addition, these differences are relatively stable when we go back further in time and almost certainly reflect the slightly higher unit costs that states initiating CON programs before 1975 tended to have.

These data are generally consistent with previous econometric findings. The presence of CON regulation rarely appears to have

Table 7.3 Expenditure Characteristics of Six Unregulated High-Cost States

States	Change in Total Expenditures (%)		Change in Cost per day (%)		Cost per Admission ($)	
	1975–1979	1973–1975	1975–1979	1973–1975	1975	1979
California	74.6	39.9	72.1	32.5	1,227	2,096
Washington, D.C.	63.9	27.3	77.9	33.7	1,431	2,724
Illinois	72.6	35.0	70.6	34.4	1,148	1,922
Michigan	68.2	40.1	67.0	28.4	1,179	1,891
Ohio	71.4	38.8	70.6	27.4	1,022	1,678
Pennsylvania	75.8	33.6	68.0	30.3	1,055	1,730
Mean	71.1	35.8	71.0	31.1	1,177	2,007
Mean, Eight Regulated States	57.8	33.8	52.3	28.9	1,225	1,849
(excluding New York)	60.8	33.8	54.1	29.0	1,168	1,798
Mean, All Other States	82.2	38.7	69.8	31.6	817	1,376

Source: Based on data from *Hospital Statistics*, various years.

a negative impact on expenditure or unit cost regressions, whether they are based on cost levels or rates of change. To the extent that CON regulation has significant impacts, they seem to increase expenditures and costs, but this effect appears to be the result of the early adoption of CON regulation in states with relatively high unit costs.

Given these simple comparative results it is worthwhile to perform more systematic statistical analyses of the expenditure and utilization experience of the hospital system, over the past eight years, with and without government regulation. We first examine a simple statistical model to determine whether government regulatory programs have had a significant effect on the growth rate of hospital expenditures, assuming that wage rates, utilization, and staffing patterns are exogenous and that the primary effects of government regulation have been to reduce organizational slack and the intensity of care available to patients admitted to the hospital. To this end, I have estimated the coefficients of the following simple expenditure growth equation for the years 1973–1979 using cross-sectional data for 50 states and the District of Columbia.

$$\text{EXPG} = A_1 + A_2\text{GAPD} + A_3\text{GWAGE} + A_4\text{GPB}$$
$$+ A_5\text{MEDICAID} + A_6\text{MEDICARE} \tag{7.1}$$
$$+ A_7\text{RATEREG} + A_8\text{CON},$$

where

EXPG = year-to-year growth rate in total hospital expenditures by state,

GAPD = year-to-year growth rate in adjusted inpatient-days by state,

GWAGE = year-to-year growth rate in average full-time equivalent employee wages,

GPB = year-to-year growth rate in personnel per bed,

MEDICAID = per capita state expenditures on Medicaid,

MEDICARE = proportion of the state's population over 65,

RATEREG = the presence of a state reimbursement regulation program. This is measured in two ways: first, as a dummy variable set equal to unity if the state had a formal rate regulation program in effect in the previous year (RATEREG1); second, as the number of years that a state had a rate regulation program in effect as of any specific year (RATEREG2).

CON = the presence of a state certificate-of-need program. It is measured in two ways, just as is the RATEREG variable (CON1 and CON2).

The empirical relationship reflects a model in which the primary factors leading to interstate differences in the rate of growth of expenditures are exogenous changes in utilization (GAPD), changes in wage rates (GWAGE), and increases in personnel (GPB). The Medicaid variable is used in an effort to measure the fiscal burden imposed on the states by Medicaid payments. The notion is that a greater burden increases the likelihood that during the past few years, states have been forced to reduce benefits or restrict reimbursements, thereby imposing some additional financial constraints on hospitals. The Medicare variable reflects the potential effects of Medicare cost reimbursement formulas on hospital expenditure behavior. These formulas discourage cross-subsidization and may make inadequate contributions for depreciation[17] and bad debts. The rate regulation variable reflects the effects of state efforts to control hospital charges, hospital reimbursement rates, and hospital budgets. The CON variable reflects the effects of capital expenditure controls on the growth in hospital costs.

If states with relatively large Medicaid burdens have tended to impose larger fiscal constraints on hospitals through the manipulation of Medicaid reimbursement policies, we expect A_5 to be negative. If Medicare reimbursement formulas, by discouraging cross-subsidization, by making more stringent allowances for depreciation, and by making it more difficult to cover bad debts, tend to have a constraining effect, we also expect A_6 to be negative. Obviously, this is a very crude measure of Medicare reimbursement contraints, and it may pick up nonregulatory factors associated with hospital utilization by the elderly. If state regulatory efforts have been successful, we expect A_7 and A_8 to be negative as well.

The estimates of equation 7.1 using ordinary least squares are reported in tables 7.4 and 7.5 for each of five years using both sets of regulatory variables. Results for the pooled data for each subperiod are also presented.

Let us consider the variables reflecting the presence of administrative regulation first (RATEREG1, RATEREG2, CON1, CON2). In all but two of the estimated equations the sign of the RATEREG variable is negative, indicating that states with administrative regulation of hospital budgets or charges have experienced lower

Table 7.4 Effects of Economic Regulation in Practice, 1973–1979 (standard errors in parentheses)

Years	Constant	GAPD	GWAGE	GPB	MEDICAID	MEDICARE	RATEREG1	CON1
1. 1979	0.15	0.51	0.022	0.076	-0.57	-0.00059	0.016	0.010
	(0.019)	(0.17)	(0.063)	(0.093)	(0.19)	(0.0015)	(0.0082)	(0.0073)
$R^2 = 0.51$								
2. 1978	0.16	0.44	0.10	0.27	-0.41	-0.0035	-0.025	0.0013
	(0.022)	(0.11)	(0.076)	(0.12)	(0.22)	(0.0017)	(0.0097)	(0.008)
$R^2 = 0.60$								
3. 1977	0.25	0.20	-0.10	-0.33	0.30	-0.007	-0.014	-0.01
	(0.027)	(0.20)	(0.15)	(0.24)	(0.31)	(0.002)	(0.014)	(0.01)
$R^2 = 0.64$								
4. 1976	0.014	0.55	0.29	0.50	-0.58	-0.0015	-0.006	0.012
	(0.024)	(0.16)	(0.073)	(0.10)	(0.24)	(0.0019)	(0.01)	(0.007)
$R^2 = 0.74$								
5. 1975–1979 (pooled)	0.19	0.60	0.095	0.19	-0.50	-0.0042	-0.018	-0.0036
	(0.014)	(0.083)	(0.039)	(0.067)	(0.15)	(0.0011)	(0.0063)	(0.0050)
$R^2 = 0.81$								
6. 1975	0.12	0.99	0.12	0.25	-0.20	0.0019	-0.011	0.004
	(0.03)	(0.13)	(0.12)	(0.18)	(0.38)	(0.0023)	(0.013)	(0.009)
$R^2 = 0.60$								
7. 1974	0.09	0.46	0.21	0.15	-0.20	0.0019	-0.008	0.004
	(0.03)	(0.14)	(0.10)	(0.15)	(0.41)	(0.0022)	(0.014)	(0.009)
$R^2 = 0.34$								
8. 1973–1975 (pooled)	0.16	0.53	-0.03	0.10	-0.45	0.00072	-0.0057	0.004
	(0.029)	(0.13)	(0.09)	(0.17)	(0.37)	(0.0022)	(0.014)	(0.004)
$R^2 = 0.18$								

Table 7.5 Effects of Economic Regulation in Practice, 1973–1979 (standard errors in parentheses)

Years	Constant	GAPD	GWAGE	GPB	MEDICAID	MEDICARE	RATEREG2	CON2
1. 1979	0.15	0.51	0.023	0.079	-0.53	-0.0006	-0.0022	0.00055
R^2 = 0.49	(0.019)	(0.17)	(0.06)	(0.09)	(0.21)	(0.0016)	(0.0013)	(0.001)
2. 1978	0.15	0.47	0.10	0.27	-0.33	-0.003	-0.005	0.0006
R^2 = 0.61	(0.021)	(0.11)	(0.076)	(0.12)	(0.22)	(0.0017)	(0.0017)	(0.0012)
3. 1977	0.24	0.86	-0.093	-0.32	0.40	-0.007	-0.0018	-0.0027
R^2 = 0.63	(0.027)	(0.21)	(0.15)	(0.25)	(0.33)	(0.0024)	(0.0029)	(0.0018)
4. 1976	0.14	0.53	0.28	0.48	-0.53	-0.0015	-0.002	-0.0006
R^2 = 0.73	(0.025)	(0.16)	(0.08)	(0.10)	(0.26)	(0.0019)	(0.0025)	(0.0016)
5. 1975–1979 (pooled)	0.19	0.61	0.09	0.19	-0.40	-0.0039	-0.003	-0.00092
R^2 = 0.46	(0.014)	(0.083)	(0.039)	(0.0067)	(0.15)	(0.0011)	(0.0012)	(0.00082)
6. 1975	0.11	1.01	0.12	0.26	-0.013	0.005	-0.004	-0.00025
R^2 = 0.60	(0.031)	(0.14)	(0.11)	(0.18)	(0.40)	(0.0023)	(0.003)	(0.002)
7. 1974	0.09	0.45	0.21	0.18	-0.37	0.002	0.002	0.0002
R^2 = 0.34	(0.03)	(0.14)	(0.10)	(0.16)	(0.46)	(0.002)	(0.004)	(0.003)
8. 1973–1975 (pooled)	0.16	0.52	-0.037	0.12	-0.69	-0.00054	0.000006	0.0024
R^2 = 0.19	(0.029)	(0.13)	(0.093)	(0.172)	(0.41)	(0.0022)	(0.0040)	(0.0024)

growth rates in total expenditures than those without such regulation. In the annual cross-sections, however, the RATEREG variables are estimated quite precisely only for the years 1978 and 1979. However, this variable is estimated with relatively small standard errors in the pooled regression equations for the 1975–1979 period.[18] There is relatively little difference in the results associated with specifying the reimbursement and CON variables as dummy variables or as variables specifying the number of years regulation has been in effect. Entering the number of years regulation has been in effect nonlinearly does not change the results significantly. On average, the presence of a state reimbursement regulation program reduced the growth in expenditures by about 10 percent over the period 1975–1979. The effect in the earlier period is not significant.

Turning next to the CON variables, we find that although the estimated coefficients are occasionally negative, they are never estimated very precisely. The estimated coefficients are insignificantly different from zero in all the pooled regressions. There has been no apparent effect of CON regulation on the growth of hospital expenditures, other things held constant.

Let us turn next to the MEDICARE variable, the proportion of the population over 65 years of age. The results here indicate that states with relatively large Medicare populations experienced a slower growth rate in expenditures during the 1975–1979 period but not during the 1973–1975 period. This result provides at least some evidence that the more formal and more stringent reimbursement formulas used by Medicare are having an increasingly important constraining effect on the financial resources available to hospitals and that they have responded by slowing the rate of growth in expenditures. However, this may also indicate that changing types of available care are being applied disproportionately to medical problems of younger patients or that they tend to be applied disproportionately in the first few days of the typical hospital stay.

Finally, consider the Medicaid variable. Recall that this variable measures the financial burden that Medicaid places on the population in a particular state. I suggested before that states with relatively generous Medicaid programs have felt increasing fiscal pressures, resulting in part from escalating Medicaid expenditures, and have responded by reducing Medicaid reimbursement rates and coverage. These actions, in turn, would place additional financial constraints on hospitals, and they would have to respond by constraining expenditure growth. The sign of the Medicaid variable is uniformly negative (except for 1977, where the entire equation yields rather peculiar results). The coefficient of the Medicaid variable is estimated quite precisely in the post-1975 period. This indicates that with utilization held constant, more stringent Medicaid eligibility and reimbursement criteria have in recent years placed significant constraints on the fiscal resources of hospitals. This has been translated into a reduction in the growth rate in hospital expenditures.

Overall the results presented here are consistent with the computations presented in tables 7.2 and 7.3. There is no statistical evidence that CON regulation independently has had any effects on hospital expenditures. Reimbursement regulation of various types appears to have significantly reduced the growth rate in expenditures, but the effects are fairly small. The indirect effects of reimbursement constraints attributable to changes in Medicaid programs and the reimbursement constraints inherent in the Medicare system also appear to have played an important role in the last few years.

The previous analysis took utilization, input prices, and staffing patterns as exogenous. Yet reimbursement and CON constraints may affect these variables directly and have more complex impacts on resource utilization than are implicit in the previous specification. To account for the potential effects of regulation on utilization, input prices, and staffing patterns, I next specify and estimate a more complex model of expenditures, utilization, input prices, and staffing patterns that also takes account of adjustment lags in these variables. The following model is specified and estimated.

$$\ln \text{EXP}_t = A_1 + A_2 \ln \text{EXP}_{t-1} + A_3 \ln \text{APD}_t + A_4 \ln \text{WAGE}_t$$
$$+ A_5 \ln \text{PBED}_t \tag{7.1}$$
$$+ A_6 \text{MEDICAID} + A_7 \text{MEDICARE}$$
$$+ A_8 \text{RATEREG} + A_9 \text{CON};$$

$$\ln \text{PBED}_t = B_1 + B_2 \ln \text{PBED}_{t-1} + B_3 \ln \text{RPCI}_t + B_4 \ln \text{INS}_t$$
$$+ B_5 \text{MEDICAID} \tag{7.3}$$
$$+ B_6 \text{MEDICARE} + B_7 \text{RATEREG} + B_8 \text{CON};$$

$$\ln APD_t = C_1 + C_2 \ln APD_{t-1} + C_3 \ln POP_t + C_4 \ln RPCI_t$$
$$+ C_5 \ln INS_t \tag{7.4}$$
$$+ C_6 MEDICAID + C_7 MEDICARE$$
$$+ C_8 RATEREG + C_9 CON;$$

$$\ln WAGE_t = D_1 + D_2 \ln WAGE_{t-1} + D_3 \ln PCI_t$$
$$+ D_4 \ln PBED_t + D_5 MEDICAID + D_6 MEDICARE$$
$$+ D_7 RATEREG + D_8 CON;$$

where

EXP_t = total state hospital expenditures in year t,
$PBED_t$ = full-time equivalent personnel per bed in year,
APD_t = adjusted inpatient-days in year t,
$WAGE_t$ = average wage per full-time equivalent employee in year t,
$RPCI_t$ = real per capita income by state in year t,
PCI_t = nominal per capita income by state in year t,
INS_t = proportion of the state population under 65 with private hospital insurance in year t,
$\ln$ = the natural logarithm of a variable,
all other variables as specified previously.

Equation 7.2 is similar to equation 7.1. It reflects the theory that equilibrium hospital expenditures are a function of utilization, input prices, and staffing patterns but that actual expenditures adjust to their equilibrium level with a lag.[19] Regulation is hypothesized to affect the equilibrium level of expenditures and perhaps the adjustment rate. Equation 7.3 reflects the theory that staffing is a function of the real income in a state and the extent of insurance coverage and that staffing patterns adjust to their equilibrium levels with a lag. We would expect the coefficients of both variables to be positive. In addition, we examine the effects of regulation on the equilibrium staffing patterns and the speed of adjustment. Equation 7.4 reflects the theory that inpatient utilization is a function of state population, real per capita income, and the extent of insurance coverage and that the utilization adjusts to its equilibrium level with a lag. We also examine the effects of regulation on utilization. Finally, equation 7.5 focuses on the wages paid to hospital workers. The hypothesis is that wages are a function of nominal per capita income and staffing patterns and that wages adjust to their equilibrium levels with a lag. The effects of the regulatory variables on wages are also analyzed. A problem with the specification used in these equations is that it assumes that adjustment rates are independent of the exogenous variables. If this is not the case, the estimates of the coefficients may confound equilibrium effects and effects on the speed of adjustment. We must therefore interpret the results with great care.

The estimates of the coefficients of this model for the period 1975–1979 using the RATEREG2 and CON2 variables are reported in table 7.6. The cross-sectional data have been pooled, and to account for the presence of a lagged endogenous variable, instrumental variables techniques have been used to generate consistent estimates. Using the RATEREG1 and CON1 variables does not change the results significantly. In light of the results for the earlier period, I report only results for the most recent period here.

The estimated coefficients of the total expenditure equation (7.2) are very similar to the results obtained for the expenditure growth equations. Reimbursement regulation has a significantly negative effect on either the equilibrium level of expenditures or the rate of adjustment in expenditures. Certificate-of-need regulation has no significant constraining effect on total hospital expenditures. The existence of a large state Medicaid burden leads to symmetrical constraints on the equilibrium level or rate of adjustment in expenditures. A large Medicare population has a similar negative effect, but it is not statistically significant. All the previous results about the effects of regulation on expenditure growth are replicated using this specification.

From equation 7.3 we see that reimbursement regulation shows no constraining effect on staffing patterns. Indeed, the estimated coefficient is positive and almost significant. Certificate-of-need regulation exhibits no significant effects, and the Medicaid burden does not appear to have had a constraining effect on either the equilibrium level of staff per bed or on the rate of adjustment. The coefficient is positive and insignificant. The only significant "regulatory" variable that appears to have any constraining effect on personnel patterns is the proportion of the population over 65. The coefficient of this variable is negative and significant. However, since elderly patients have relatively high average lengths of stay, this may very well reflect differences in optimal staffing patterns for longer-stay patients rather than the effects of reimbursement constraints. It is difficult to disentangle these two potential causal relationships. The negative sign of the real income

Table 7.6 The Effects of Regulation on Hospital Expenditures, Input Prices, and Utilization, 1975–1979 (standard errors in parentheses)

(7.2) $\ln \text{EXP}_t = -3.02 + 0.39 \ln \text{EXP}_{t-1} + 0.61 \ln \text{APD}_t + 0.76 \ln \text{WAGE}_t + 0.35 \ln \text{PBED}_t - 1.63 \text{ MEDICAID}$
      (0.29)   (0.055)   (0.055)   (0.07)   (0.052)   (0.31)

      $- \, 0.0016 \text{ MEDICARE} - 0.11 \text{ RATEREG2} + 0.0038 \text{ CON2}$
      (0.0023)   (0.0023)   (0.0016)

      $R^2 = 0.99$

(7.3) $\ln \text{PBED}_t = 0.76 + 0.41 \ln \text{PBED}_{t-1} - .0021 \ln \text{RPCI}_t + 0.53 \ln \text{INS}_t + 1.29 \text{ MEDICAID} - 0.016 \text{ MEDICARE}$
      (0.35)   (0.32)   (0.00066)   (0.20)   (0.97)   (0.0074)

      $+ \, 0.012 \text{ RATEREG2} - 0.00053 \text{ CON2}$
      (0.007)   (0.0018)

      $R^2 = 0.70$

(7.4) $\ln \text{APD}_t = 0.15 + 1.04 \ln \text{APD}_{t-1} - 0.042 \ln \text{POP}_t - 0.0035 \ln \text{RPCI}_t + 0.26 \ln \text{INS}_t - 1.13 \text{ MEDICAID}$
          $(0.041)\,(0.075) \qquad (0.075) \qquad\qquad (0.0044) \qquad\qquad (0.016) \qquad (0.38)$

          $\phantom{\ln \text{APD}_t =} - 0.0068 \text{ MEDICARE} - 0.00084 \text{ RATEREG2} + 0.0018 \text{ CON2}$
          $\phantom{\ln \text{APD}_t =} (0.0049) \qquad\qquad (0.0021) \qquad\qquad (0.0013)$

$R^2 = 0.99$

(7.5) $\ln \text{WAGE}_t = 0.32 + 0.97 \ln \text{WAGE}_{t-1} - 0.01 \ln \text{PCI}_t - 0.036 \ln \text{PBED}_t + 0.10 \text{ MEDICAID} - 0.0035 \text{ MEDICARE}$
          $(0.81)\,(0.21) \qquad\qquad (0.14) \qquad (0.05) \qquad\qquad (0.39) \qquad (0.0021)$

          $\phantom{\ln \text{WAGE}_t =} + 0.0013 \text{ RATEREG2} - 0.0016 \text{ CON2}$
          $\phantom{\ln \text{WAGE}_t =} (0.0024) \qquad\qquad (0.0015)$

$R^2 = 0.89$

variable is surprising. Other things equal, we would expect higher per capita incomes to lead to greater demands for high-quality hospital care, which in turn should lead to a greater number of hospital staff per bed. It is likely that this variable is picking up differences in the rates of adjustment in staffing between high-income and lower-income states. This is consistent with the suggestion that lower-income states may be catching up with the frontier hospital care provided in the high-income areas. There is also some evidence that the extent of hospital insurance affects the level of staffing and associated availability of high-quality medical care, as we would expect.

Let us turn next to the utilization equation (7.4). There is no significant statistical evidence that either reimbursement regulation or certificate-of-need regulation has affected hospital utilization as measured by the number of days of inpatient-care. The state Medicaid burden seems to have led to reduced hospital utilization. Whether this effect falls entirely on the poor or, through its effects on hospital budgets, leads to more general constraints on hospital admissions or length of stay cannot be determined from the available aggregate data. The Medicare variable also indicates a constraining effect, although it is not statistically significant. Here, however, we can be more confident that we are picking up an effect of stringent reimbursement rather than an effect that is essentially demographic, as in equation 7.3. Other things equal, we would expect inpatient-days to be higher in states with a larger elderly population. The negative coefficient estimated for this variable gives some support to the hypothesis that federal Medicare reimbursement constraints have led hospitals to curtail utilization. As with the Medicaid effect, we have no way of knowing whether this constraint affects primarily the elderly, or through the budgetary constraints on hospitals, leads to more restrictive utilization policies. The population variable and the per capita income variable are not significantly different from zero, although the insurance variable is positive and significant, as we would expect. It appears that this specification is not picking up the full complexities of the dynamics of utilization over this period.

Finally, let us consider the wage equation. There is little evidence that any of the regulatory variables have had any effect on the equilibrium level or adjustment rate of wages, except perhaps for the Medicare variable. Indeed, the only variables that have any predictive power for this year's wages are last year's wages and the number of personnel per bed. Here again it appears that wages are adjusting much more slowly in the heavily staffed areas than in the areas with less staff per bed and presumably less sophisticated care. Again, this is consistent with the catching-up hypothesis.

This more detailed exploration of the effects of economic regulation on hospital facilities and reimbursement adds little to what we already know. There appears to be a general constraining effect on the equilibrium level and/or adjustment rate of hospital expenditures provided by various forms of reimbursement constraint. No such constraining effects can be identified for certificate-of-need regulation alone. When we focus on the effects of regulation on specific measurable components of hospital expenditures, the results are not particularly revealing. There is no evidence that either formal reimbursement regulation by independent commission or certificate-of-need regulation has constrained the number of inpatient-days, personnel per bed, or wages. There is some evidence that more stringent reimbursement and coverage rules for Medicaid patients in states with historically generous Medicaid programs have led to a reduction in inpatient utilization. Similar but more ambiguous results may be associated with Medicare.

How then have reimbursement constraints led to the observed reduction in the growth rate of hospital expenditures? A number of hypotheses are consistent with the data. First, we would expect any binding budgetary constraint to lead hospitals to improve management techniques in order to eliminate organizational slack and encourage more efficient provision of care. Second, binding budget constraints may lead hospitals to consolidate certain facilities and to engage in more joint activities. Both of these would represent largely one-shot savings. Third, hospitals may be saving money by reducing the utilization of inpatient diagnostic and therapeutic techniques and by introducing new ones more slowly. The aggregate data on days of care and on personnel that we have used so far do not allow us to determine this. Fourth, there is some weak evidence that reimbursement constraints resulting from more stringent Medicaid and Medicare reimbursement criteria have led to a reduction in inpatient utilization. Finally, the observed reduction in the growth rate of expenditures may be due more to the greater prevalence of regulation in states with

sophisticated systems and to a reduction in the rate of technological change "on the frontier," which is exogenous to the system,
than to regulation, although data presented in table 7.3 do not
lend much support to this theory. It also seems clear that New
York is an outlier and has applied more stringent constraints having more readily observable effects on the supply of facilities and
the utilization of hospitals.

Case Study: The Discussion of CT Scanners

Most empirical efforts to assess the effects of government regulation on hospital expenditures, input utilization, and patient utilization are based either on aggregate cross-sectional data by state
on variables such as total expenditures, expenditures per day,
total hospital beds, and personnel per bed or on similar variables
obtained for a cross section of individual hospitals. Given the
previous results, such data make it difficult to pinpoint regulatory
impacts. A better understanding of both hospital behavior and
performance and the effects of government regulation requires an
examination of much more disaggregated data on the services
offered by hospitals and the extent to which they are utilized. If
the major source of real increases in hospital expenditures is the
introduction of new services and increases in the intensity with
which both new and existing services are used, the long-term
effectiveness of regulatory programs must depend on constraints
on the rate of introduction and utilization of specific diagnostic
and therapeutic modalities. As a result, it would be extremely
useful to analyze the effects of government regulation on specific
types of services and facilities.

The earliest planning and regulatory efforts associated with
certificate-of-need regulation focused on the supply of general
hospital beds. This is the only area in which empirical research
has identified a significant constraint imposed by certificate-of-
need regulation. In many states attention to general hospital beds
naturally led to an examination of obstetrical bed supplies and in
some cases to the supply of specialized pediatric beds.[20] More
recently, considerable attention and controversy has been associated with the rapid introduction of CT scanning equipment.[21]
CT scanners were introduced commercially in the United States
in 1973 and spread among hospitals quickly. Over 1,200 CT scanners now operate in the United States, and nearly 1,000 hospitals

have either a head scanner, a whole body scanner, or both. The CT scanner has become, for many critics of the American hospital system, a symbol of what is bad about technological change. The federal government and state planning and CON agencies have promulgated guidelines for the purchase of CT scanners, and this new technology is usually identified as a prime candidate for regulatory constraint.[22] The vast majority of CT scanners in the United States were installed while CON regulation and reimbursement regulation were in place in many states. It therefore seems useful to examine the effects that administrative regulation has had on the introduction of CT scanning equipment as a case study of regulatory effectiveness.

We would expect the number of CT scanners in any state, in equilibrium, to reflect the aggregate demand for CT scanning services and any constraints on supplying all the services demanded that might be imposed by government regulation. Aggregate demand would, in turn, be a function of variables such as the size of the population, per capita income, population density, and extent of insurance coverage. Using cross-sectional data for the number of CT scanners operating in each state as of February 1979, I have estimated the following simple linear regression model to assess the effects of administrative regulation on the diffusion of CT scanners:

$$\ln \text{SCAN} = A_1 + A_2 \ln \text{POP} + A_3 \ln \text{PCI} \qquad (7.6)$$
$$+ A_4 \ln \text{PD} + A_5 \text{RATEREG} + A_6 \text{CON},$$

where

SCAN = number of CT scanners (head + body) in each state as of February 1979,[23]
POP = state population in 1978,
PCI = per capita state income in 1978,
PD = population density,
RATEREG = one of two variables indicating the existence or age of a formal state reimbursement regulation program; RATEREG1 and RATEREG2,
CON = one of two variables indicating the existence or age of a state certificate-of-need program; CON1 and CON2,
$\ln (x)$ = the natural logarithm of variable x.

I expect states with larger populations and higher per capita incomes to have higher aggregate demands for CT scanning services. States with relatively low population densities should have higher aggregate demands to compensate for the longer distances patients would otherwise have to travel, holding population and income constant. Thus we expect A_2 and A_3 to be positive and A_4 to be negative.

To the extent that certificate-of-need agencies have been successful in using their permit authority to constrain hospitals from introducing CT scanners, we would expect A_6 to be negative. If these agencies have not imposed binding constraints on hospital decisions to install CT scanners, A_6 should be zero. Similarly, if binding budgetary constraints have led hospitals to defer the rate of growth in CT scanning services, we would expect A_5 to be negative; if financial constraints have not led hospitals to defer CT scanners, A_5 would be zero.

There is an important difference between these two types of constraints. To the extent that CON agencies have had an effect on the number of CT scanners installed, they have probably done so through the direct use of their planning and permit authority. The effects of binding budget constraints would be more indirect. By providing more general financial constraints, the regulatory agency gives individual hospitals more freedom to allocate scarce resources as they see fit. If, at this stage of the diffusion process, hospitals view additional CT scanning facilities as representing relatively low valued uses of resources, we would expect them to respond to budget constraints by limiting the allocation of resources to additional CT scanners. If, on the other hand, additional facilities are viewed as having relatively high net benefits, we may observe little or no effect on the number of CT scanning facilities. At this stage of the diffusion process hospitals may respond to binding budget constraints by reducing resource utilization in other areas perceived to represent smaller sacrifices in net benefits.

The estimated values for the coefficients of equation 7.6 for both variants of the regulatory variables are the following (standard errors are in parentheses):

$$\ln \text{SCAN} = -18.1 + 1.05 \ln \text{POP} + 1.4 \ln \text{PCI} - 0.03 \ln \text{PD}$$
$$\phantom{\ln \text{SCAN} = } (4.0) \quad (0.06) \qquad (0.45) \qquad (0.04)$$

$$\phantom{\ln \text{SCAN} = } -0.22 \text{ RATEREG1} - 0.11 \text{ CON1,}$$
$$\phantom{\ln \text{SCAN} = } (0.15) \qquad\qquad (0.14)$$

$R^2 = 0.89.$

$$\ln \text{SCAN} = -17.4 + 1.05 \ln \text{POP} + 1.3 \ln \text{PCI} - 0.01 \ln \text{PD}$$
$$\quad\quad (3.8) \quad (0.06) \quad\quad\quad (0.42) \quad\quad\quad (0.04)$$

$$-0.05 \text{ RATEREG2} - 0.004 \text{ CON2},$$
$$(0.028) \quad\quad\quad (0.02)$$

$R^2 = 0.89$.

Consider the demand variables first. State population is, not surprisingly, an important determinant of the number of CT scanners installed across states. The estimated coefficient, which can be interpreted as an elasticity, is not significantly different from unity. State per capita income is also a significant determinant of the number of CT scanning facilities. The estimated elasticity is also not significantly different from unity. The elasticity of the number of scanners with respect to income is, I believe, surprisingly high, probably because CT scanners have not yet "saturated" the system and because hospitals in more affluent states have tended to introduce them more rapidly. The coefficient of the population density variable is negative, as expected, but it is not estimated very precisely. I believe that this too reflects a technology that is still being rapidly diffused through the system. Any effort to freeze the acquisition of additional CT scanning facilities would be a disadvantage to low-income states and would keep states with low population densities from installing additional facilities to compensate for longer average travel distances.

In all cases the regulatory variables have negative signs, but only the rate regulation coefficient is estimated with any reasonable degree of precision. In addition, in the first formulation rate regulation has twice the impact of CON regulation, and in the second formulation it has ten times the impact of CON regulation. On average the presence of rate regulation in a state reduces the number of CT scanners operating by about 20 percent.

CT scanners may be installed in hospitals and in physicians' offices, and administrative regulation may affect the location of CT scanners in a variety of ways. Stringent rate regulation applied only to hospitals may lead physicians to substitute office-based facilities for hospital-based facilities. Similarly, since few CON agencies have authority over office facilities, restrictions on permits for hospital-based CT scanners might lead to a substitution of office-based facilities. On the other hand, both physicians and hospitals must convince third-party payers that reimbursement should be allowed for particular services. One of the reasons that hospital associations have supported CON regulation is that need "certified" by a government agency virtually assures reimbursement. Thus in a state with a CON regulation program that is not restrictive but serves primarily as an administrative permitting authority, physicians may find it more desirable to use hospital-based facilities, which carry with them greater certainty of reimbursement. Stringent regulation of either kind applied to hospitals should tend to lead to a substitution of office-based facilities for hospital-based facilities. However, if CON regulation merely provides a certification mechanism that insures reimbursement, facilities may be more likely to be located where the certification can be obtained—in hospitals.

I am reluctant to attach normative significance to any observed substitution of office-based CT scanners for hospital-based CT scanners. To the extent that such substitutions are made possible by the incomplete reach of hospital regulation, such responses may be viewed as a way of circumventing efforts to constrain the total supply of such facilities. On the other hand, this type of substitution may be quite desirable from a cost-effectiveness perspective because it may result in a commensurate substitution of lower-cost outpatient care for higher-cost inpatient care. Thus we may consider one objective of hospital regulation to be a desire to shift some patient care from an inpatient basis to an outpatient basis to conserve resources. Appropriate data to analyze this issue further are not available.

To explore effects of administrative regulation on the location of CT scanners, we examine variations in the proportion of CT scanners located in physician offices across states as explained by differences in per capita income, population density, and the extent of government regulation. The following linear regression equation was estimated:[24]

$$\text{SCANP/SCAN} = A_1 + A_2\text{PCI} + A_3\text{PD} \qquad (7.9)$$
$$+ A_4\,\text{RATEREG} + A_5\,\text{CON},$$

where SCANP is the number of CT scanners in physicians' offices and all other variables are as previously defined.

The ordinary least-squares estimates of equation 7.9 are the following (standard errors are in parentheses):

$$SCANP/SCAN = 0.17 + 0.000005 \text{ PCI} - 0.000002 \text{ PD}$$
$$\qquad\quad (0.17) \quad (0.00002) \qquad\quad (0.00002)$$
$$+ 0.15 \text{ RATEREG1} - 0.09 \text{ CON1,}$$
$$\qquad (0.056) \qquad\qquad (0.052)$$
$$R^2 = 0.15;$$

$$SCANP/SCAN = 0.018 - 6 \times 10^{-7} \text{ PCI} - 0.000006 \text{ PD}$$
$$\qquad\quad (0.17) \quad (0.00002) \qquad\quad (0.000006)$$
$$+ 0.027 \text{ RATEREG2} - 0.008 \text{ CON,}$$
$$\qquad (0.01) \qquad\qquad (0.0076)$$
$$R^2 = 0.14$$

These results, along with the previous results, add a number of interesting conclusions. The only variables in equation 7.9 with any significant explanatory power are the regulatory variables. The ceofficients of the rate regulation variables are consistently positive and are estimated fairly precisely. The coefficient of the CON variables are negative but are estimated much less precisely. The previous results indicated that the only significant constraint on the total supply of CT scanners in particular states appeared to be rate regulation. These additional statistical results indicate that reimbursement constraints may also lead to a substitution of office-based CT scanners for hospital-based CT scanners, partially offsetting some of the impact of hospital regulation on the total supply of CT scanners but perhaps also achieving cost savings by increasing the proportion of CT scanning done on an outpatient basis. On the other hand, although there is little evidence that CON regulation affects the total supply of CT scanners, there is some evidence that in states with CON regulation such facilities are more likely to be located in hospitals than in physicians' offices. This result may be explained by the value of a certificate of need for assuring reimbursement in states that have such procedures. This may have undesirable cost consequences if the net effect is that patients who could just as well be treated on an outpatient basis at lower total cost are treated on an inpatient basis.

This simple exploration leads to conclusions that are consistent with the rest of the discussion in this chapter. Rate or reimbursement regulation once again appears to represent a binding financial constraint to which hospitals must respond. In the case of CT scanners they respond by installing a smaller number of such facilities and by substituting office-based facilities for hospital-based facilities. There is little evidence that CON regulation has affected the supply of CT scanners. To the extent that there is any effect, it appears to be to increase the attractiveness of hospital-based utilization, and this may lead to higher costs rather than lower costs.

Conclusions

In summary, all the empirical evidence to date supports the conclusion that massive certificate-of-need apparatus has had little effect on hospital expenditures and utilization. There is some evidence that CON regulation affects the supply of general hospital beds, but similar results have not been replicated for ancillary services or total expenditures. The largest effects of economic regulation that have been identified are associated with government efforts to control hospital expenditures directly using budget review procedures and reimbursement formulas based on normative criteria. These regulatory efforts appear to have had some success in imposing binding financial constraints that have forced hospitals to curtail the growth rate of expenditures. New York has gone the furthest in this direction. Most other states that have used reimbursement controls have applied them more gradually and less severely. While these other states have not experienced the dramatic reductions in expenditure growth that New York has, they also have not had to encounter the enormous provider and community opposition that has characterized the squeeze in New York. Whether these efforts can continue in the long run without causing severe constraints on the quantity and quality of care is not yet known. Most of the states identified as successful in controlling the growth in hospital expenditures are high-cost states offering intensive hospital services. It may be much easier to apply modest constraints to these hospital systems than to those that are still catching up.

The Role of Government Regulation

There is general agreement that the hospital system in the United States is characterized by costly inefficiencies. There is considerably less agreement about the specific magnitude of these inefficiencies and how these inefficiencies are distributed between resource expenditures that provide no value to patients and those that provide some value but at levels substantially below the social opportunity cost of the resources utilized. There is substantial disagreement about the appropriate direction for public policies aimed at ameliorating the inefficiencies that characterize the demand and supply of hospital care under prevailing institutional arrangements.

State and federal policy to control hospital expenditures has been predicated on the assumption that economic regulation can achieve cost containment goals effectively and efficiently. Yet the theoretical and empirical evidence on economic regulation in this sector indicates that many of the regulatory instruments that have been employed have not been very effective. At worst, these programs entail substantial administrative expenses while promising little effect on resource expenditures and utilization or even perverse effects. At best, we can expect moderate improvements in resource allocation and quantitatively significant reductions in hospital expenditures compared with the status quo. But the improvements are likely to be much less significant than many of the proponents of economic regulation would lead us to believe. The fundamental difficulty with all the proposed regulatory programs is that they deal with symptoms rather than causes.

However, it is impossible to evaluate the desirability of economic regulation in a vacuum. We must compare the various forms of economic regulation to the alternatives. Furthermore, we must determine which forms of economic regulation are likely to perform best if public policy continues to take this direction. Among the plethora of public policy suggestions for reform, economic regulation appears to be the only policy response that has captured any degree of political consensus.

In comparing economic regulation to the alternatives, we must first compare it with the status quo. If the alternative is to rely on existing institutional arrangements for determining the demand, supply, and financing of hospital care, are we better off with government regulation or are we better off allowing the system to operate without additional regulatory constraints? I believe that some economic regulation is better than nothing and that particular forms of economic regulation dominate others. I also believe that we must have limited expectations for what even the most effective types of economic regulation can actually achieve when we consider the inherent imperfections of even the most attractive forms and the political constraints.

Since the prevailing system is characterized by many performance failures, economic regulation does not have to deal with all the real and perceived problems in order to be desirable. Economic regulation is inherently imperfect, but so is the prevailing system. Economic regulations that are likely to improve the performance of the hospital system may be worth pursuing, especially if the chosen regulatory instruments do not preclude more fundamental changes.

I believe that some form of reimbursement constraint on individual hospitals seems likely to improve the allocation of resources to and within the hospital system and is superior to other regulatory programs that have been initiated or considered. I am especially attracted to the use of general budget constraints of the type described in chapter 6. This form of economic regulation has the greatest prospect for encouraging hospitals to utilize resources more efficiently and to reduce the growth rate in hospital expenditures. It is the only form of economic regulation that has actually had even limited effectiveness.

The Carter administration's proposed cost containment programs are prototypes of such economic regulation. The general approach taken by the Carter administration made good sense and, in principal, could have provided efficient incentives to hospitals to reduce expenditures and improve resource allocation. However, I believe that the proposals had several problems that can and should be remedied. First, the proposals tried to do too much too soon. The implied constraints on real expenditure growth indicated by the formulas were much too large and would have been applied too quickly. They would have imposed a very severe constraint on a dynamic system with considerable inertia and without appropriate decision processes to allocate scarce resources efficiently. I suspect that the size of the constraint and the speed with which it would have been applied was heavily influenced by the administration's interest in balancing the federal budget for fiscal year 1981. Second, the Carter administration's proposal was completely insensitive to the diversity among hospitals within states and between hospitals in terms of the types of patients treated and the diffusion of state-of-the-art medical technology. It tried to apply uniform growth rate constraints to a system without base-level uniformity in any relevant dimension. The diversity in the hospital system must be given at least some recognition in any regulatory strategy. Third, the original proposals included redundant and possibly distortionary restrictions on capital expenditures to include the planning-CON system in the program. Both the capital restrictions and much of the planning-CON system are unnecessary and possibly counterproductive.

To work well and have a reasonable prospect for obtaining a political consensus, general reimbursement constraints must initially be less severe than those proposed by the Carter administration and should be tightened only as the system adapts to them and as we accumulate experience with the results. A more modest constraint would be a more desirable start than a constraint that implies a rapid cut of 75 percent in real expenditure growth. Furthermore, because of the great diversity among hospitals and across states I believe that the federal government is not the proper level for applying these constraints. The states are in a better position to impose budgetary constraints to reflect prevailing demand and supply characteristics. The states have at least two incentives to initiate reimbursement or budget constraint programs. First, the states must bear a large fraction of the increasing Medicaid expenditures. Second, they inevitably face political pressure to limit increases in private insurance premiums. Given the limited diffusion of mandatory state reimbursement regulation programs, however, these incentives do not appear to have been sufficient to encourage most states to implement such programs. Since a substantial fraction of the financial burden of hospital expenditures falls on the federal government, in the form of Medicare and Medicaid payments and tax subsidies to private insurance, efforts would have to be made to internalize these burdens to the states by giving them some additional incentives to implement budget constraint programs. For example, the federal government could announce general targets for reducing the real rate of growth in hospital expenditures compared with some base period and split the expenditure savings (adjusted for inflation) with the states. The funds would be returned to the states in the form of general revenues to be used in any way the state pleases. The federal government could provide additional funds to help pay for setting up state reimbursement regulation programs.

This approach gives the states broad financial incentives to contain hospital costs, beyond any prevailing incentives. Individual states would then be free to decide whether they want to regulate, how they will regulate, and the severity of the constraint that is most appropriate for the state as a whole and for individual hospitals. The states would be free to institute regulatory programs such as those in New York and Maryland or to pursue other appropriate means for containing costs. The federal government merely provides the incentives to contain costs and additional financial help to finance reimbursement regulation programs if the states choose to use them. A state that believed it had a more effective way to contain costs would be free to use it and would still receive a share of the savings. States that felt that prevailing supply and demand conditions did not justify expenditure constraints would also be free to do nothing and forego the direct and "shared" benefits of cost containment. My expectation is that under prevailing institutional arrangements the incentives will lead many additional states to institute reimbursement control programs similar to those used elsewhere.

Certificate-of-need regulation has serious theoretical shortcomings, promises relatively little in the way of savings, and has yielded no identifiable savings where it has been utilized. I feel that the federal government should stop encouraging the growth of CON regulation and should shift federal funds from the planning-CON apparatus to state reimbursement regulation programs. Whatever useful elements of the planning apparatus exist should be integrated into the reimbursement regulation process. Our long experience with planning-CON regulation indicates that it is a failure. There is little reason for the federal government to promote it when superior regulatory instruments are available.

An attractive characteristic of a regulatory program based on broad, state-implemented budgetary constraints is that it does not impede more fundamental changes that may be occurring naturally or may be encouraged by additional public policy initiatives.

The states would have additional incentives to encourage the development of less expensive competing health plans and to encourage third-party payers to develop independent reimbursement constraints. Binding budget constraints would encourage hospitals to become affiliated with health maintenance organizations that constrain hospital admissions and to cooperate with third-party payers in developing additional financial incentives to reduce the demand for care by patients and physicians. Perhaps most important, of course, hospitals would face financial incentives to eliminate organizational slack and facility duplication and to ration marginal care. As long as the budget constraints imposed are not too severe, serious adverse selection problems in which high-cost patients are improperly turned away from hospitals would not arise.

We should be realistic about what can be achieved by this type of regulatory program. I believe that real savings can be achieved with modest administrative costs and without severe sacrifices in the quality of care. However, I do not believe that the enormous savings projected by the Carter administration can be achieved by reimbursement regulation. While the states may be able to tighten the budget constraints as such a program evolves, our medium-term expectations must be fairly modest. The regulatory constraints that we are applying are imperfect and are being applied in a system in which the relevant agents face very limited independent incentives to conserve resources. We are treating the symptoms the best way that we can, but we are not dealing with the underlying sources of the resource allocation problems in the hospital system.

While some economic regulation may be better than nothing, ideally we would like to deal directly with the underlying causes of resource misallocation. There is no theoretical reason that the alternative to economic regulation is the status quo. Many economists have suggested changes in prevailing institutional arrangements that would restore economic incentives to conserve resources and promote price competition. The most recent articulation of a scheme to make the market work better is due to Enthoven.[1] He envisions a system in which consumers are given incentives to choose freely among alternative health care delivery systems on the basis of cost as well as quality. He anticipates that appropriate incentives will lead to the development of different types of prepaid group practices and alternative health delivery plans, not tied to the workplace, as feasible alternatives to the prevailing fee-for-service, cost-based third-party reimbursement system. He believes that appropriate incentives to individuals will lead to a market for health care delivery in which market competition is an effective regulator of the quantity, quality, and costs of health care. He expects such a system to yield approximately the same quality of care at substantially lower costs. Furthermore, the health care system that will emerge as a consequence of fair economic competition will be fundamentally different from the present system and will rely much more heavily on competing HMOs and much less on fee-for-service, cost-based third-party reimbursement.

Enthoven paints such an optimistic picture of the prospects for a health care system based on freedom of choice and market competition that it is worth exploring the policy changes necessary to bring it about. He presents several broad principles for promoting "fair economic competition" in the health care system. First, he suggests that each year all consumers should be given the opportunity to enroll in any approved health plan operating in their area with traditional fee-for-service, third-party insurance offered as one of the choices. Second, he argues that any subsidies provided for purchasing health insurance or for paying for enrollment in an HMO should be fixed in dollar terms for any individual. Thus the dollar subsidy provided to any individual would be the same whether he chose a high-cost or a low-cost plan so that the subsidies would not distort choices among competing plans. However, these subsidies could vary among individuals. The poor and the elderly, for example, would get more than young, affluent individuals. Third, all competitors would have to adhere to the same rules regarding eligibility for enrollment, premium computations, and minimum standards for services covered. Enthoven would require all plans to have periods of open enrollment and would severely limit experience rating to avoid adverse selection problems. Finally, Enthoven suggests that physicians should be organized in competing economic units so that the premium each group charged would reflect its cost experience. It is unclear whether Enthoven means to require physicians to join prepaid group practices or sees this as the likely outcome of a competitive market system. I assume that it is the latter.

I have little doubt that the combination of mandated choice and nondistortionary fixed-dollar subsidies will promote more economic competition among insurance and alternative health delivery plans. The first is already a federal requirement for firms with more than 25 employees in areas with qualified HMOs. The second, however, will require substantial changes in the tax laws and the ways in which we pay for Medicaid and Medicare enrollees. There is little reason to dwell on the enormous political problem entailed in making such changes, so let us assume that this can somehow be accomplished. Even given these changes I am much less optimistic than Enthoven about the results.

First, the proposed program has a substantial regulatory component to it. Enthoven requires that all plans have open enrollment and use modified community rating rather than experience rating. He also requires that plans provide specified minimum coverages. It is easy to write a law that requires firms to serve all on an equal basis and to refrain from experience rating. It is much harder to enforce such restrictions because it is not in the interest of competitive firms to adhere to them. Competing firms will still be able to compute the true actuarial risks associated with different individuals and groups of individuals and will have enormous incentives to avoid serving those with unattractive risk characteristics, given the premiums established by community rating. There are numerous subtle ways to evade such restrictions in the pursuit of lower costs and higher profits. It is also easy to write minimum coverages into an insurance contract; but if competing insurance plans can profit by evading the minimums, enforcement may be a substantial task. Therefore, it seems that this program is still likely to need government regulation to ensure that competing health plans adhere to restrictions that are not in their interest. Of course, the costs of such regulation may be worth incurring.

Second, while I find the HMO experience encouraging, I am reluctant to accept the extrapolations that have been made to the entire hospital system. Our experience with HMOs is limited and has evolved under the umbrella of the prevailing fee-for-service, cost-based reimbursement system. There are substantial self-selection biases in the patient populations served by HMOs and in the physician population that has chosen to practice in HMOs. Many HMOs appear to have performed well, but there have also been many examples of HMOs that have performed poorly. I believe that HMOs and alternative delivery systems should be given a fair chance to compete with the fee-for-service, cost-based reimbursement system. However, I find little in the available data to predict the ultimate saturation rates of these organizations or their ultimate cost savings.

Third, it is not obvious that many areas of the country can sustain a sufficient number of alternative health plans to ensure effective competition. HMOs appear to be characterized by significant economies of scale.[2] Our experience to date is that entry is far from easy and that it can take many years for an HMO to attain a significant market penetration. These factors, combined with the limited number of secondary and tertiary care facilities in many areas of the country, at least raise the possibility that many markets will be characterized by duopoly or oligopoly behavior and performance rather than anything approaching pure competition. At best, given the substantial quality dimension in health care, we are talking about markets that are monopolistically competitive, with all the ambiguous welfare properties that market equilibrium in such situations may imply.[3] Furthermore, even in the best of worlds, it will take many years for competing delivery systems to develop. As of mid 1980 fewer than 40 qualified HMOs were operating in the entire country. It is not clear that duopoly or oligopoly will yield market outcomes very much different from what we already have in many areas of the country. Indeed, despite the substantial market saturation achieved by Kaiser in California, the competitive fee-for-service sector has one of the highest average costs per admission in the country.

To the extent that effective competition has been restricted as a result of provider power, linkages between providers and insurers, advantages provided to Blue Cross, and refusals to deal, such restrictions will at the very least retard the development of competing plans engendered by improved incentives. Any public policy initiatives in the health care system, whether they be oriented to increasing competition or based on some form of incentive-based regulation, must include provisions for eliminating any residual restrictions on free competition in these markets. These provisions should include a reevaluation of the applicability of the antitrust laws to health insurers and health care providers, especially exemptions that may be provided by the McCarran-Ferguson Act. Any monopolistic behavior that can be constrained by antitrust sanctions should be vigorously pursued. Unfortunately, antitrust powers are most limited in duopoly and oligopoly situations, where conscious parallel behavior is possible without explicit agreements to restrain trade. This may be the market structure that will emerge in many areas.

Despite these potential problems, many of the reforms suggested by Enthoven and others make good sense. They will almost certainly lead to improvements in the allocation of resources in the health care system generally and in the hospital system in particular. I hope that they can be implemented. However, the magnitude of the savings that will be realized is uncertain, and the government will have to continue to play a substantial role as a regulator of competing health plans and as a redistributor of income. Furthermore, the full benefits of whatever competition may eventually emerge will take many years to be realized, because profound changes in the delivery system will be required to sustain the outcomes that Enthoven believes are possible.

If there is a reasonable prospect that reforms such as these can be enacted over the next few years, is there still a role for reimbursement regulation based on general binding budget constraints? I believe that the answer is yes, at least for a transitional period. Even if we are very optimistic about the prospects for these fundamental reforms, there is likely to be considerable interest in containing hospital expenditures during the transitional period, which may be very long. General budget constraints, implemented by the states, represent the best regulatory alternative for getting from here to there. Such constraints provide incentives for hospitals to develop mechanisms for allocating scarce resources, which will be needed even when fundamental reforms are eventually achieved. They can yield real resource savings during the transitional period and may encourage hospitals to develop health maintenance organizations and other alternatives. Furthermore, general budget constraints can provide a backstop in areas in which effective competition does not emerge. Finally, if we can replace certificate-of-need regulation with reimbursement regulation based on general budget constraints, we will eliminate what may prove to be a significant barrier to fundamental change. If alternative public policy initiatives are successful in containing hospital expenditures as advertised, the kinds of binding budget constraints that I have suggested would become redundant and the system could easily be scrapped.

My enthusiasm for economic regulation of the hospital system is far from overwhelming. Our general experience with economic regulation in this country over the past couple of decades, combined with the complexities and peculiarities of the hospital system, must lead any prudent economist to recommend more government regulation only with great caution. Yet out system is so riddled with imperfections and inefficiencies and is placing such a large financial burden on the economy that imperfect regulation is likely to be better than nothing. The fundamental changes that may ultimately ameliorate the causes of resource misallocations still appear to be a long way off, and they do not represent a realistic short-run alternative. Furthermore, we have already embarked down the road of economic regulation of hospitals in this country, but the heavy emphasis on planning and certificate-of-need constraints has been ill advised. Economic regulation that uses modest but binding general budget constraints is certainly superior to the existing planning-CON process. So I conclude that there is a useful role for government regulation in the hospital sector and that we can identify specific regulatory instruments that are most likely to be productive. I believe that we should make prudent use of these instruments with full recognition of their inherent limitations and the difficulties that they will encounter in practice.

Notes

Chapter 2

1. This book focuses on nonfederal short-term general hospitals, often called acute or community hospitals. Hospital care is also provided in federal hospitals (military, Veteran's Administration, Public Health Service) and in long-term care facilities. Acute-care hospitals have different economic characteristics than either federal or long-term care facilities and treat different types of patients. It is the acute-care hospitals that have been the focus of state and federal regulatory interventions. Except where noted, all data are for nonfederal short-term general hospitals.

2. For a comprehensive survey of the economic literature on government regulation see Joskow and Noll (1981).

3. See *Hospital Statistics 1980* (Chicago: American Hospital Association, 1980), pp. 191–204.

4. Ibid., pp. 20–141.

5. Ibid., pp. 20–141.

6. See *Social Security Bulletin Annual Statistical Supplement*, pp. 12–14, U.S. Department of Health and Human Services, Social Security Administration, September 1980 (Washington, D.C.: U.S. Government Printing Office) and "Ten Years of Short-Stay Hospital Utilization and Costs under Medicare: 1967–76," Health Care Financing Administration, August 1980 (HCFA-03053).

7. See Davis and Schoen (1978).

8. Depending on what price index one uses to deflate the expenditure data.

9. Good hospital input price indexes are not available for years prior to 1970.

10. Input price changes are almost certainly not independent of changes in factor input utilization. As a result this estimate is probably a lower bound for the true cost of increased intensity.

11. The automation of various clinical laboratory procedures falls in this category. Open-heart surgery falls in the second category. CT scanning has characteristics of both a product and a process innovation. See Fineberg et al. (1977) and Bartlett et al. (1978).

12. National Academy of Sciences (1979), Rabkin and Melin (1978), Russel (1979), Altman and Blendon (1979), Wagner and Zubkoff (1978).

13. Reports prepared by the AHA Hospital Administrative Services contain a detailed breakdown of the costs incurred by a large sample of community hospitals in providing services in specific cost and revenue centers within hospitals. These data provide a rare opportunity to obtain

a picture of cost and utilization by diagnostic, therapeutic, and nursing service units within the hospital.

14. In 1979 over 3,000 community hospitals had diagnostic radioiosotope facilities while only 900 had CT scanners. See *Hospital Statistics 1980,* American Hospital Association, pp. 203–204.

15. Open-heart surgery is discussed in more detail in Schwartz and Joskow (1980a).

16. This dynamic process is nicely documented by Julianne Howell in "Regulating Hospital Capital Investment: The Experience in Massachusetts" (Ph.D. thesis, John F. Kennedy School of Government, Harvard University, 1980).

Chapter 3

1. See statement of Joseph Califano in *Health Cost Containment,* Hearings before the Subcommittee on Health of the Committee on Finance, U.S. Senate, 96th Congress, March 13, 1979.

2. See Arrow (1976) and Zeckhauser (1970).

3. Ibid.

4. I do not like the term *moral hazard* as used in this context. There is certainly nothing immoral about following incentives to consume additional hospital care. Nevertheless, this is the term used in the insurance literature. The efficiency loss often associated with moral hazard is also problematical. In a sense the welfare loss attributed to moral hazard is a lower-bound estimate of the transactions costs associated with implementing an ideal contract. Incurring these transactions costs would not improve welfare.

5. Barzel (1980) has done some interesting work examining the characteristics of private insurance contracts.

6. For example, Enthoven (1978, 1980) seems to focus on these kinds of ex post comparisons.

7. See Feldstein (1971, 1973, 1977), Feldstein and Freidman (1977), and Pauly (1979).

8. Mitchell and Phelps (1976).

9. See Wagner and Zubkoff (1978) and National Academy of Sciences (1979).

10. J. E. Harris (1979b).

11. The types of services available at a point in time to any individual are a function of the extent of insurance coverage in the community generally, other things equal.

12. It is well known that markets will not provide every variety or quality of a product that consumers are willing to pay for when there are some economies of scale in production. When there is quality competition and

substitute products, a "minority" product quality is less likely to be produced. See Spence (1976).

13. Pauly (1979).

14. Based on Harris (1979b), footnote 8, which takes account of individuals with no insurance.

15. Zeckhauser (1979), p. 39.

16. Hospitals normally have a set of posted charges, which include a charge per day for basic care and separate charges for particular ancillary services. However, the largest third-party payers often negotiate a separate reimbursement arrangement based on accounting procedures designed to determine the average costs incurred by the patients for which individual third-party payers are responsible.

17. Less than half of the Blue Cross plans use cost-based reimbursement, but these plans are concentrated in the most populous states. See Weiner (1977) for a general discussion of reimbursement policies.

18. The Social Security Amendments of 1972, PL 92-603, introduced certain reasonableness and comparative cost criteria. See Weiner (1977).

19. In 1976 the largest commercial insurer accounted for less than 4 percent of total health insurance reimbursements. Each of the top ten commercial insurers accounted for, on average, 2 percent of reimbursements. Blue Cross and Blue Shield account for about 50 percent of reimbursements.

20. See Frech and Ginsburg (1978).

21. This does not mean that incentive contracts cannot be conceptualized. See Newhouse and Taylor (1971). They just are not being made available in the current market environment.

22. The literature on hospital objective functions and associated hospital behavior is extensive. See, for example, Newhouse (1970), Davis (1972), and Pauly and Redisch (1973).

23. See Joskow (1980).

24. Ibid.

25. See J. E. Harris (1977).

26. Recent financial pressures resulting from reimbursement regulation and changes in Medicare and Medicaid reimbursement policies in a world of rapid inflation have begun to lead to some organizational changes.

27. J. E. Harris (1979a).

28. When patients choose to insure themselves by participating in a health maintenance organization (HMO), they may be making this kind of implicit contract. HMOs are organized to give physicians cost containment incentives. They also provide comprehensive inpatient and outpatient coverage so that any financial biases toward inpatient care from the patient's perspective are eliminated. The major difference between HMO enrollees and comparable groups of individuals is that HMO enrollees have lower hospitalization rates and greater use of ambulatory services. See Luft (1978).

29. *Argus Charts*, National Underwriter Company (Cincinnati).

30. Anderson (1975), Law (1974), Hetherington et al. (1975) Eilers (1963).

31. Law (1974), p. 19.

32. Frech and Ginsburg (1978), Berman (1978), Robbins (1978).

33. See also Kass and Pautler (1979).

34. Berman (1978).

35. See *American Medical Association v. U.S.*, 317 U.S. 519 (1943), 110 F.2d 703.

36. For example, Douglas and Miller (1974). See also Joskow (1980).

37. Feldstein (1971, 1973, 1977), Feldstein and Friedman (1977), and Pauly (1979).

38. Ibid.

39. See Feldstein and Friedman (1977).

40. See J. E. Harris (1979b).

41. See Bunker (1970), Lembke (1952), Wennberg (1975), and Gaus, Cooper, and Hirschman (1976), Fuchs (1974), chapter 2.

42. See, for example, Doyle (1953), Trussel et al. (1962), Morton et al. (1968).

43. Moore (1978), Rutkow and Zuidema (1978), New York Medical Society (1970, 1972), and Emerson (1976).

44. This approach was used in a much cited congressional study, *Surgical Performance: Necessity and Quality*, U.S. Congress, House Committee on Interstate and Foreign Commerce, Subcommittee on Oversight and Investigations, 85th Congress, 1978.

45. These issues are discussed in Schwartz and Joskow (1980b). The observation that physicians disagree on the appropriate course of treatment does not mean that one is clearly right and the other wrong. Conflicting medical evidence and uncertainty leads to considerable diversity in "good care." We certainly cannot conclude that a recommendation for surgery is wrong just because a consulting physician disagrees.

46. Abrams (1979) and Eisenberg et al. (1977).

47. See, for example, Bartlett et al. (1978), Fineberg et al. (1977), and Wortzman et al. (1975).

48. McClure (1976).

49. Finkler (1979).

50. Schwartz and Joskow (1980a).

51. Statement of Honorable Joseph A. Califano, Secretary of Health, Education, and Welfare, in "President's Hsopital Cost Containment Proposal," Joint Hearing before the Subcommittee on Health of the Committee on Ways and Means and the Subcommittee on Health and the Environment of the Committee on Interstate and Foreign Commerce, U.S. House of Representatives, March 12, 1979 (serial 96-18), p. 16.

52. The origins and justification of these "ideal" ratios are obscure. Their use seems to go back to the start of the Hill-Burton hospital construction programs.

53. A number of the issues discussed later are treated in more detail in Joskow (1980) and Schwartz and Joskow (1980a).

54. B. Clark and A. Lamont, "Accurate Census Forecasting Leads to Cost Containment," *Hospitals*, June 1, 1976, pp. 21–22.

Chapter 4

1. The area's aggregate demand function may cross the average cost function in a range of increasing returns.

2. For example, the demand function for some service may fall entirely below the average cost function characterized by declining unit costs. This means that there is no single price at which the service can break even. Although there is not a single price at which this service can be economically provided, the total value of the service to patients may still be greater than the total costs. If price discrimination among patients were possible, the hospital might be able to generate sufficient revenues to cover total costs. For a multiproduct hospital, the alternative to price discrimination across patients would be cross-subsidization via price discrimination across services. Situations of this sort that may arise in a market characterized by product variety and monopolistic competition are discussed by Spence (1976).

3. Thus no effort is made to account for the so-called Roemer effect, which implies that supply somehow creates demand. The theoretical foundations for this proposition are virtually nonexistent, and the empirical observations on which it is based are consistent with alternative models of market behavior that do not depend on the assumption that physicians maintain unexploited power to increase the demand for care. See Shain and Roemer (1959), Newhouse (1974), and Newhouse (1978), p. 55.

4. In short, it is assumed that the physician does not consider the relationship between the care provided to individual patients, aggregate hospital costs, and the associated level of insurance premiums that all purchasers of insurance must pay.

5. Presumably insurance premiums would be reduced enough in the long run to compensate for the reduction in the care that is available in certain circumstances when an individual becomes ill.

6. See Peltzman (1973) and Grabowski (1975).

7. Patients and physicians may perceive larger differences than can be supported by the available scientific evidence. Furthermore, even if the differences are small or zero, physicians are likely to resist changes in their well-established modes of practice, and insured patients are unlikely to give up anything they perceive as being beneficial. In many circum-

stances patients may perceive that medicine can do more for them than it really can. It is unlikely that such perceptions will change quickly. As a result, we can expect substantial discontent with mandatory reductions in the quantity and quality of care that can be made available.

8. See Luft (1978).

9. See Cooper (1975).

10. See Culyer (1976).

11. This in turn will depend on the magnitude of the supply constraint and the ways in which available resources are rationed. If it is true that on the margin health care resources are associated with very small expected benefits, and the marginal care can be effectively rationed, patients would not perceive any significant reduction in the quality of care.

12. Thus an individual who voluntarily joins an HMO may understand that the lower cost of care, reflected by his insurance premium and negligible coinsurance rate, is associated with some restrictions on how much care will be provided and who will provide it when he becomes ill. On the other hand, an individual who has chosen a conventional private insurance plan without any implied restrictions on the availability of care, does not expect to be told that he cannot be hospitalized promptly (for example) because patients with a greater need are ahead of him on a long queue.

13. Averch and Johnson (1962).

14. Sheshinski (1971).

Chapter 5

1. To meet minimum federal standards a CON program must have a threshold of no more than $150,000. Many states have established lower thresholds.

2. The National Health Planning and Resource Development Act of 1974, January 4, 1975: 88 STAT. 2225.

3. Lewin and Associates (1974).

4. The historical evolution of certificate-of-need regulation has been well documented by Havighurst (1974). Here I provide only a brief summary.

5. Gottlieb (1974), p. 11.

6. Ibid.

7. Lave and Lave (1974) and U.S. Department of Health, Education, and Welfare (1975).

8. Lave and Lave (1974), pp. 2–8.

9. Curran (1974), p. 5.

10. Gottlieb (1974), p. 19.

11. In short, they had an interest in capturing the process and using it for their own benefit.

12. On average, capital costs account for less than 10 percent of total expenditures (interest plus depreciation divided by total expenditures). This figure can be inferred from data reported by the Hospital Administrative Survey. If public programs account for 50 percent of total expenditures, the exposure is likely to be quite small.

13. In 1979 I made a request to HEW for information on the number of projects that had been denied reimbursement under this authority. I was told that such information has never been compiled.

14. Lewin and Associates (1974).

15. PL 96-641 (January 4, 1975), Section 1523(4).

16. Ibid., Section 1521 (2)(C)(4)(d).

17. Health Planning and Resource Development Amendments of 1979 (PL 96-79), 93 STAT. 592.

18. 42 CFR 121.

19. 42 CFR 123 (E).

20. Havighurst (1973).

21. This simply requires that hospitals would not be joint profit maximizers if they could collude effectively because they value the scope and intensity of care that each of them individually can deliver.

22. See Luft et al. (1979).

23. National Guidelines for Health Planning, 42 CFR 121.1–121.6, 121.201–121.211.

24. For example, the Commonwealth of Massachusetts has developed its own standards for facilities such as CT scanners, intensive and coronary care units, and general acute-care beds.

25. See, for example, Bicknell and Walsh (1975) and Bicknell and Van Wyck (1979).

26. CT scanners, open-heart surgery and cardiac catheterization, therapeutic radiology, and general hospital beds.

27. Joskow (1973).

28. Policy Analysis, Inc. (1980).

29. Applied Management Sciences (1978), Evans and Jost (1978), Martin (1972), Warner (1979).

30. For example, hospitals could satisfy average occupancy rate guidelines by delaying discharges and increasing the average length of stay.

31. Havighurst (1973) and Posner (1974), p. 115.

32. Schwartz and Joskow (1980a).

33. Proposed Hospital Cost Containment Act of 1977 (HR 6575) *Congressional Record*, April 25, 1977 p. H3527. A revised bill introduced in 1979 did not have a capital investment ceiling (S570, 96th Congress, first session). The capital expenditure ceiling was included in the Carter admin-

istration's national health insurance proposals (proposed National Health Plan Act HR 5400, 96th Congress, first session).

34. We can also think of it as reflecting a concern about the so-called Roemer effect and related agency problems.

35. See J. E. Harris (1977, 1979a).

36. Issues such as this are partially responsible for the opposition to the Carter administration's cost containment proposals among rural congressmen and congressmen representing communities with relatively less sophisticated and costly hospital care.

37. Curran (1974), p. 88.

38. Policy Analysis, Inc. (1980).

39. Havighurst (1973), pp. 1173–1188.

40. Joskow (1980).

41. American Hospital Association (1977b), McMahon (1979).

42. Lewin and Associates (1974), p. 210.

43. American Hospital Association (1977b).

44. Fitzpatrick (1979), p. 30.

45. Policy Analysis, Inc. (1980).

46. Cohodes (1979), p. 30.

47. PL 86-641 (January 4, 1975), Section 1521 (2)(C)(4)(d).

48. Cohodes (1979), pp. 17–28, and Lewin and Associates (1974).

49. Ibid.

50. See Policy Analysis, Inc. (1980).

51. Criteria have been established for general hospital beds, CT scanning facilities, intensive and coronary care facilities, diagnostic radiology facilities, laboratories, and ambulatory care facilities.

52. A compilation of these legislative efforts to override CON decisions was obtained from the Massachusetts Department of Public Health for the period through 1979.

53. Bicknell and Walsh (1975).

54. Bicknell and Van Wyck (1979).

55. These figures are based on a compilation of all decisions made regarding acute hospitals during this period, which was done at my request by Michael Salinger.

56. In several cases approval was granted for only a portion of the request.

57. See Alvin Headen, "Measuring the Effects of Economic Regulation: Certificate-of-Need Regulation of Hospitals in Massachusetts 1972–1978," Ph.D. dissertation, Massachusetts Institute of Technology, 1981.

58. The Harbridge House (1979) study of the costs and benefits of CON regulation in Massachusetts takes this approach. Focusing on capital costs "deterred" is not likely to yield a useful benefit measure.

Chapter 6

1. That is, the explicit terms of the insurance contract as represented by the coinsurance provisions and the kinds of services covered do not change. The implicit terms of the insurance contract, of course, do change if supply constraints lead to excess demand and the system cannot supply all the care that would otherwise be demanded given the explicit terms of the contract.

2. These programs are discussed further later in this chapter.

3. See Lewin and Associates (1974) and American Hospital Association (1977b). It appears that many Blue Cross plans have become much more active in trying to constrain hospital expenditures and utilization. This may reflect increasing difficulties in getting insurance premium increases accepted by state insurance commissions. See Harry Schwartz, "Health Insurance: A Fight for Survival," *New York Times,* October 20, 1977, p. 3F; "New Blue Shield Policies Stir Protests from Michigan M.D.'s," *American Medical News,* September 19, 1977; Dolores Katz, "State Wants Grip on Hospitals, Blues," *Detroit Free Press,* July 27, 1977, p. 1.

4. "Jersey Hospitals Go from Time Clock to Piece Work," *New York Times,* April 27, 1980, p. 6E. For a detailed discussion of this type of program, see "A Prospective Reimbursement System Based on Patient Case-Mix for New Jersey Hospitals, 1976–78," *Health Care Financing* (Research and Demonstration Series) Report No. 3, Department of Health, Education, and Welfare, 1978.

5. See Cohen (1978).

6. See Garfield and Lovejoy (1964) and Kahn (1970).

7. For example, Joskow (1974).

8. The extent of cross-subsidization in a multiproduct firm is difficult both to define and to measure. The conventional wisdom seems to be that outpatient, obstetric, and pediatric inpatient facilities are money losers while laboratories and radiology departments are money makers. On May 1, 1980, the Massachusetts Rate Setting Commission proposed new regulations which would, among other things, preclude cross-subsidization. This proposed regulation, along with others that would reduce reimbursement for Medicare and Medicaid patients, have been vigorously opposed by the hospitals in Massachusetts. See "Open Letter to Governor King," *Boston Globe,* June 22, 1980, p. 43.

9. J. Harris (1979) suggests otherwise, but his idea is to develop rate structures that depart from costs to achieve a second-best optimum in the face of low coinsurance rates. The problem is that many patients with cost-based insurance policies never really see the posted charges.

10. This is essentially what Medicare and other cost-based reimbursement plans do.

11. See Sattler (1976) and Bauer (1978).

12. A retrospective system that used stringent utilization criteria for reimbursement could be much more effective than a prospective budget that allows the hospital great latitude in making cost and utilization projections.

13. See, for example, Lave et al. (1972). The comparable-hospital approach was incorporated in the second version of the Carter administration's cost containment bill (S570, 1979).

14. See Lave and Lave (1978).

15. Hospitals falling below the regression line may be allowed to keep some of the difference as an incentive. However, we can anticipate that nonprofit hospitals will find some way to spend the surplus.

16. Of course, fixing the production set at a point in time could provide a rather stringent constraint. I think that it makes more sense to think of this in the context of the formula approach discussed later.

17. New York has adopted a formula approach. See Berry (1976) and discussion later in this chapter.

18. Needless to say there is also enormous controversy over the appropriate normative criteria to use regarding both cost considerations and efficacy considerations. I am always amazed at how quickly policymakers accept particular judgments that support a policy when a fair reading of the clinical literature clearly indicates considerable uncertainty and often profound disagreements. The discussion of unnecessary surgery is one of the worst examples of this phenomenon.

19. The Carter administration's cost containment proposal changed in response to congressional opposition. The simplicity that characterized the original proposal was replaced with much more complexity, involving more regulation by the Secretary of Health and Human Services.

20. The evolution of the Carter administration's proposals is itself evidence of this tendency to create an increasingly complicated formula.

21. For example, the 1979 version of the Carter administration's cost containment bill added comparable-hospital criteria that did not exist in the original version of the bill.

22. Joskow (1974).

23. See the papers compiled in Hamilton (1979).

24. This adjustment is sometimes made retrospectively, however, so that the effects of regulatory lag would be associated only with underestimates of input price inflation. See Worthington, Tyson, and Chin (1979).

25. See Cohen (1978) for a discussion of regulatory lag in Maryland.

26. These plans are often voluntary only in the sense that hospitals can decline to participate if they are willing to forego reimbursement by Blue Cross.

27. Fitzpatrick (1979).

28. The following discussion draws heavily on Hamilton and Kamens (1979), General Accounting Office (1980), and private communications.

29. See Joskow (1974) and Joskow and MacAvoy (1975) for a discussion of the effects of regulatory lag and regulatory commission behavior as it has affected electric utilities in an inflationary world.

30. The following discussion draws heavily on Weinstein and DeMarco (1979), General Accounting Office (1980), material made available to me by the Massachusetts Rate Setting Commission, and private communications.

31. This discussion draws heavily on Hamilton, Weinstein, and Lee (1979), General Accounting Office (1980), and private communications.

32. *Modern Health Care*, September 1977, p. 20.

33. Davis and Schoen (1978), chapter 3.

34. "Hospitals Feel Pinch of Medicaid Cuts," *Boston Globe*, April 16, 1978; "Direct Correlation between High Welfare Loads, Low Operating Margins," *Hospitals*, March 1, 1977; "Medical Squeeze: Health Insurance Plans Are Forcing Hospitals to Impose Economies," *Wall Street Journal*, June 21, 1977. See Stuart (1976).

35. See Weiner (1977) and W. Cleverly, "Is Hospital Capital Being Eroded under Cost Reimbursement?" *Hospital Administration*, Summer 1974, pp. 58–73. The use of straight-line depreciation based on original cost does not adequately account for the effects of inflation on replacement costs of capital equipment.

36. *Congressional Record*, April 25, p. H3527 (HR 6575).

37. "The Hospital Cost Containment Act of 1977: An Analysis of the Administration's Proposal," prepared by the Congressional Budget Office, June 1977, (Washington, D.C. U.S. Government Printing Office, 1977).

38. See the statements of the representatives of these groups in "President's Hospital Cost Containment Proposal," Joint Hearing before the Subcommittee on Health of the Committee on Ways and Means and the Subcommittee on Health and the Environment of the Committee on Interstate and Foreign Commerce, U.S. House of Representatives, May 1977, part 1 (Serial 95-20) and part 2 (Serial 95-21).

39. David Stockman and Phil Gramm "The Administration's Case for 'Hospital Cost Containment': A Critical Analysis," May 16, 1979 (mimeographed).

40. *Congressional Record*, March 6, 1979, p. H1106.

41. Statement of Honorable Joseph Califano in "President's Hospital Cost Containment Proposal," Joint Hearing before the Subcommittee on Health of the Committee on Ways and Means and Subcommittee on Health and the Environment of the Committee on Interstate and Foreign Commerce, House of Representatives, 96th Congress, first session, March 1979, part 1 (Serial 96-18), p. 18.

42. It is interesting to compare the "waste" estimated in the 1977 hearings with similar estimates presented in the 1979 hearings. The savings at-

tributed to excess beds increased by a factor of 2, for example. The HEW estimates of "waste and inefficiency" appear to have been pulled out of a hat. Stockman and Gramm, "Case for 'Hospital Cost Containment,' " provide an interesting and amusing commentary.

Chapter 7

1. Salkever and Bice (1976).

2. Hellinger (1976).

3. Sloan and Steinwald (1980).

4. Joskow (1980).

5. Policy Analysis, Inc. (1980).

6. Hellinger (1978) also observed this phenomenon.

7. Policy Analysis, Inc. (1980), table 4.1, Fitzpatrick (1979), and Fallon (1979).

8. The Health Insurance Plan of Greater New York (HIP) had 770,000 members in 1978. *National HMO Census of Prepaid Group Plans* (1978). U.S. Department of Health, Education and Welfare, Office of Health Maintenance Organizations (Rockville, Maryland).

9. Ibid.

10. Most of this decline occurred before 1979. The rate of decline slowed considerably in 1979, and one wonders whether New York has gone about as far as it can.

11. "Pact on Hospitals Signed: Koch-Harris Feud Ends," *New York Times*, June 25, 1980, p. B1; "U.S. Acts to Block Closing of Sydenham," *New York Times*, May 15, 1980; Fallon (1979).

12. "Care at Many Hospitals Hit Sharply by Cutbacks," *New York Times*, May 13, 1980, p. B1; "Hospital in Brooklyn to Accept State Aid," *New York Times*, May 14, 1978, p. 32.

13. There is no easy way to distinguish between the two. My impression from what I have learned about the New York experience is that reimbursement controls represent the binding regulatory constraint. Additional evidence reported next supports this view.

14. See notes 11 and 12.

15. The difference in means is statistically significant at the 1 percent level.

16. Once we recognize that the opportunity set is expanding as a result of technological change and that the rate and direction of technological change are at least partially exogenous, the reduction in the growth rate of expenditures in states that are on the "frontier" may be explained by a reduction in the rate of expansion of that frontier.

17. See discussion in chapter 6.

18. I have also estimated "smoothed" regression equations which use the

total growth rate in expenditures in each time period as the independent variable rather than using year-by-year observations. For example, for the period 1975 to 1979 we have

GEXP = 0.45 + 1.09 GAPD + 1.08 GWAGE − 1.16 MEDICAID
         (0.13)   (0.22)   (0.19)   (0.84)

        − 0.015 MEDICARE − 0.018 RATER + 0.003 CON2,
        (0.0065)   (0.0084)   (0.0032)

$R^2 = 0.79$,

where RATEREG2 and CON2 take their 1976 values. The results are qualitatively the same as those reported in the text.

19. The underlying specification of the model is a "rigidity model." For example, assume that equilibrium expenditures (EXP_t^*) are given by

$$\text{EXP}_t^* = A_1 + A_2 \text{APD}_t + A_3 \text{RATEREG},$$

but that adjustment to the equilibrium is gradual

$$(\text{EXP}_t - \text{EXP}_{t-1}) = \gamma (\text{EXP}_t^* - \text{EXP}_{t-1}); \quad 0 < \gamma < 1.$$

Using the first expression and rewriting the second, we get

$$\text{EXP}_t = \gamma A_1 + \gamma A_2 \text{APD}_t + \gamma A_3 \text{RATEREG} + (1 - \gamma) \text{EXP}_{t-1}.$$

Alternatively, we can think of a model in which the regulation variables affect the speed of adjustment to a new equilibrium but not the equilibrium itself. For example, we might have

$$\text{EXP}_t^* = A_1 + A_2 \text{APD}_t,$$

$$(\text{EXP}_t - \text{EXP}_{t-1}) = \gamma(1 + k \text{RATEREG})(\text{EXP}_t^* - \text{EXP}_{t-1}).$$

This leads to a much more complex expression in which regulatory variables enter linearly as before and interactively. The interpretations of the coefficient estimates would also necessarily be different. I have not reported the results from more complex specifications of this basic model here. However, in discussing the effects of the regulatory variables, I indicate that the estimated coefficients may be subject to alternative interpretations.

20. Federal standards for the supply of obstetrical services and pediatric inpatient services were established in 1978. 42 CFR 121.203, 121.205–121.206.

21. See "Policy Implications of the Computed Tomography (CT) Scanner," Office of Technology Assessment, U.S. Congress, August 1978, and "CT Scanners: A Technical Report," American Hospital Association (1977).

22. See, for example, the Statement of Joseph Califano, secretary of Health, Education and Welfare, Congressional Hearings (1979), p. 16.

23. Data were obtained from the Office of Technology Assessment. Approximately two-thirds of the scanners were installed after June 1976. The rate of growth in CT scanner installations appears to have slowed in the last year or two. As of early 1979 all but 16 HSAs had at least one CT scanner.

24. Including other independent variables such as population or the number of radioisotope facilities does not affect the basic results.

Chapter 8

1. Enthoven (1980).

2. See, for example, "Health Maintenance Organizations Can Help Control Health Care Costs," General Accounting Office (PAD-8–17), Washington, D.C., May 6, 1980, Appendix I.

3. See Spence (1976).

Bibliography

Abrams, H.
1979
"The 'Overutilization' of X-Rays." *New England Journal of Medicine* 300:1213–16.

Altman, S. H., and R. J. Blendon, eds.
1979
Medical Technology: The Culprit behind Health Care Costs? Proceedings of the 1977 Sun Valley Conference on Health Care. Washington, D.C.: Department of Health, Education, and Welfare.

American Hospital Association
1977a
CT Scanners: A Technical Report. Chicago.

American Hospital Association
1977b
Hospital Regulation: Report of the Special Committee on the Regulatory Process. Chicago.

Anderson, O.
1975
Blue Cross since 1929: Accountability and the Public Trust. Cambridge, Mass.: Ballinger.

Anderson, R., and O. Anderson
1967
A Decade of Health Services. Chicago: University of Chicago Press.

Applied Management Sciences
1978
A Feasibility Study of the Influence of Capital Expenditures on Hospital Operating Costs, Final Report. Washington, D.C.: Health Care Financing Agency, Research and Demonstration Series #6.

Arrow, K.
1976
"Welfare Analysis of Changes in Health Coinsurance Rates." In R. Rosett, ed., *The Role of Health Insurance in the Health Services Sector.* New York: National Bureau of Economic Research.

Averch, H., and L. Johnson
1962
"Behavior of the Firm under Regulatory Constraint." *American Economic Review* 52:1053–69.

Bartlett, J., et al.
1978
"Evaluating Cost-Effectiveness of Diagnostic Equipment: The Brain Scanner Case." *British Medical Journal* 2:815–820.

Barzel, Y.
1980
"Competitive Tying Arrangements," Mimeographed. September.

Bauer, K. G.
1978
"Hospital Ratesetting—This Way to Salvation?" In M. Zubkoff et al., eds., *Hospital Cost Containment: Selected Notes for Future Policy*. New York: Prodist.

Berry, R. E.
1976
"Prospective Rate Reimbursement and Cost Containment: Formula Reimbursement in New York." *Inquiry* 13:288–301.

Bicknell, W. J., and D. C. Walsh
1975
"Certificate-of-Need: The Massachusetts Experience." *New England Journal of Medicine* 292:1054–61.

Bicknell, W. J., and J. Van Wyck
1979
"Certificate-of-Need: The Massachusetts Experience, January 1974–June 1979." Mimeographed.

Bunker, J.
1970
"Surgical Manpower: A Comparison of Operations and Surgeons in the United States and England and Wales." *New England Journal of Medicine* 282:135–144.

Bunker, J., and J. Wennberg
1973
"Operation Rates, Mortality Statistics, and the Quality of Life." *New England Journal of Medicine* 289:1249.

Calabresi, G., and P. Bobbit
1978
Tragic Choices. New York: Norton.

Cohen, H. A.
1978
"Experiences of a State Cost Control Commission." In M. Zubkoff et al., eds., *Hospital Cost Containment: Selected Notes for Future Policy*. New York: Prodist.

Cohodes, D. C.
1979
"The State Experience with Capital Management and Capital Expenditure Review Programs." Urban Systems Research and Engineering. Mimeographed.

Commonwealth of Massachusetts
1976
"Proposal in Response to Request for Proposal #SSA-76-0127 For Type II Development Contract." Rate Setting Commission. January 15.

Cooper, M. H.
1975
Rationing Health Care. New York: John Wiley & Sons.

Culyer, A. J.
1976
Need and the National Health Service. Totowa, N.J.: Rowman and Littlefield.

Curran, W. J.
1974
"A National Survey and Analysis of State Certificate-of-Need Laws for Health Facilities." In C. C. Havighurst, ed., *Regulating Health Facilities Construction. Washington, D.C.: American Enterprise Institute.*

Davis, K.
1972
"Economic Theories of Behavior in Nonprofit Private Hospitals." *Economic and Business Bulletin* 24:1–13.

Davis, K., and C. Schoen
1978
Health and the War on Poverty: A Ten-Year Appraisal. Washington, D.C.: Brookings.

Douglas, G. W., and J. C. Miller
1974
Economic Regulations of Domestic Air Transport. Washington, D.C.: Brookings.

Dowling, W. L.
1974
"Prospective Reimbursement of Hospitals." *Inquiry* 11:163–180.

Doyle, J.
1953
"Unnecessary Hysterectomies." *Journal of the American Medical Association* 151:360.

Eisenberg, J. M., et al.
1977
"Computer-Based Audit to Detect and Correct Overutilization of Laboratory Tests." *Medical Care* 15:915–921.

Emerson, R.
1976
"Unjustified Surgery, Fact or Myth?" *New York State Journal of Medicine* 76:454.

Enthoven, A. C.
1980
Health Plan. Reading, Mass.: Addison-Wesley.

Enthoven, A.
1978
"Shattuck Lecture—Cutting Cost without Cutting the Quality of Care." *New England Journal of Medicine* 298:1229–38.

Evans, R., and R. Jost
1978
"Economic Analysis of Body Computed Tomography Units Including Data on Utilization." *Radiology* 127:151.

Fallon, J.
1979
Statement on Behalf of the National Conference of State Legislators during Hearings on the President's Hospital Cost Containment Proposal before the Subcommittee on Health of the Committee on Ways and Means, U.S. House of Representatives, 96th Congress, March 23, 26, 29 (No. 96-19).

Feldstein, M. S.
1971
"Hospital Cost Inflation: A Study of Non-Profit Price Dynamics." *American Economic Review* 61:835–872.

Feldstein, M. S.
1973
"The Welfare Loss of Excess Health Insurance." *Journal of Political Economy* 81:251–280.

Feldstein, M. S.
1977
"Quality Change and the Demand for Hospital Care." *Econometrica* 45:1681–1702.

Feldstein, M. S., and B. Friedman
1977
"Tax Subsidies, the Rational Demand for Insurance, and the Health Care Crisis." *Journal of Public Economics* 7:155–78.

Fine, J., and M. Morehead
1971
"Study of Peer Review of Inhospital Patient Care." *New York State Journal of Medicine* 71–84.

Fineberg, H., et al.
1977
"Computerized Cranial Tomography: Effect on Diagnostic and Therapeutic Plans." *Journal of the American Medical Association* 238:224–227.

Finkler, S.
1979
"Cost Effectiveness of Regionalization: The Heart Surgery Example." *Inquiry* 16:264–270.

Fitzpatrick, J. H.
1979
Statement on Behalf of the Hospital Association of New York State during Hearings on the President's Hospital Cost Containment Proposal before the Subcommittee on Health of the Committee on Ways and Means, U.S. House of Representatives, 96th Congress, March 23, 26, and 29 (Serial 96-19).

Frech, H. E., and P. G. Ginsburg
1978
"Competition among Health Insurers." In *Competition in the Health Care Sector: Past, Present, and Future.* Washington, D.C.: Federal Trade Commission, March.

Fuchs, V.
1974
Who Shall Live? New York: Basic Books.

Garfield, P. J., and W. F. Lovejoy
1964
Public Utility Economics. Englewood Cliffs, N.J.: Prentice-Hall.

Gaumer, G., et al.
1979
"Prospective Reimbursement in Connecticut." *Topics in Health Care Financing* 6:52–57.

Gaus, C., B. Cooper, and C. Hirschman
1976
"Contrasts in HMO and Fee-for-Service Performance." *Social Security Bulletin.* 39:3–14.

General Accounting Office
1980
"Rising Hospital Costs Can Be Restrained by Regulating Payments and Improving Management." (HRD-80-72). Washington, D.C.: U.S. Government Printing Office, September 19.

Goldberg, L., and W. Greenberg
1978
"The Emergence of Physician-Sponsored Health Insurance: A Historical

Perspective." In W. Greenberg, ed., *Competition in the Health Care Sector.* Washington, D.C.: Federal Trade Commission.

Gottlieb, S.
1974
"A Brief History of Health Planning in the United States." In C. Havighurst, ed., *Regulating Health Facilities Construction.* Washington, D.C.: American Enterprise Institute.

Grabowski, H.
1975
Drug Regulation and Innovation. Washington, D.C.: American Enterprise Institute.

Hamilton, D., and G. Kamens
1979
"Prospective Reimbursement in New York." *Topics in Health Care Financing* 6:96–107.

Hamilton, D., R. Weinstein, and A. J. Lee
1979
"Prospective Reimbursement in Washington State." *Topics in Health Care Financing* 6:117–126.

Harbridge House, Inc.
1979
"An Inquiry into the Costs and Benefits of the Massachusetts Determination of Need Program." Boston.

Harris, J. E.
1977
"The Internal Organization of Hospitals: Some Economic Implications." *Bell Journal of Economics* 8:467–482.

Harris, J. E.
1979a
"Regulation and Internal Control in Hospitals." *Bulletin of the New York Academy of Medicine* 55:88–103.

Harris, J. E.
1979b
"The Aggregate Coinsurance Rate and the Supply of Innovations in the Hospital Sector." Mimeographed.

Harris, J.
1979
"Pricing Rules for Hospitals." *Bell Journal of Economics* 10:224–243.

Havighurst, C. C.
1973
"Regulation of Health Facilities and Services by 'Certificate-of-Need.' " *Virginia Law Review* 59:1143–1232.

Hellinger, F. J.
1976
"The Effect of Certificate-of-Need Legislation on Hospital Investment."
Inquiry 13:187–193.

Hellinger, F. J.
1978
"An Empirical Analysis of Several Prospective Reimbursement Systems."
In M. Zubkoff et al., eds., *Hospital Cost Containment: Selected Notes for
Future Policy*. New York: Prodist.

Hetherington, R. W., et al.
1975
Health Insurance Plans: Promise and Performance. New York: John Wiley
& Sons.

Joskow, P. L.
1973
"Pricing Decisions of Regulated Firms: A Behavioral Approach." *Bell
Journal of Economics and Management Science* 4:118–140.

Joskow, P. L.
1974
"Inflation and Environmental Concern: Structural Change in the Process
of Public Utility Price Regulation." *Journal of Law and Economics* 17(2):291–327.

Joskow, P. L.
1980
"The Effects of Competition and Regulation on Hospital Bed Supply and
the Reservation Quality of the Hospital." *Bell Journal of Economics*
11(2):421–447.

Joskow, P. L., and P. MacAvoy
1975
"Regulation and the Financial Condition of the Electric Power Companies
in the 1970s." *American Economic Review* 65:295–301.

Joskow, P. L., and R. Noll
1981
"Regulation in Theory and Practice: An Overview." In G. Fromm, ed.,
Studies of Public Regulation. Cambridge, Mass.: MIT Press.

Kahn, A. E.
1970
The Economics of Regulation. Vol. 1: Principles. New York: John Wiley.

Kahn, A. E.
1979
"Applications of Economics to an Imperfect World." *American Economic
Review* 69:1–13.

Kass, D., and P. Pautler
1979
Staff Report on Physician Control of Blue Shield Plans. Washington, D.C.: Federal Trade Commission, November.

Lave, J., and L. Lave
1978
"Hospital Cost Function Analysis: Implications for Cost Controls." In M. Zubkoff et al., eds., *Hospital Cost Containment: Selected Notes for Future Policy.* New York: Prodist.

Lave, J., and L. Lave
1974
The Hospital Construction Act: An Evaluation of Hill Burton Programs, 1948–1973. Washington, D.C.: American Enterprise Institute.

Lave, J., et al.
1972
"Hospital Cost Estimation Controlling for Case Mix." *Applied Economics* 4:165–180.

Law, Sylvia
1974
Blue Cross: What Went Wrong? New Haven, Conn.: Yale University Press.

Lembcke, P.
1952
"Measuring the Quality of Medical Care through Vital Statistics Based on Hospital Service Areas, I: Comparative Study of Appendectomy Rates." *American Journal of Public Health* 42:276–286.

Lembcke, P.
1967
"Evolution of the Medical Audit." *Journal of the American Medical Association* 199:543–550.

Lewin and Associates, Inc.
1974
"Nationwide Survey of State Health Regulations." Prepared for the Health Resources Administration: HRA-OC-75-002. September.

Lewis, C.
1969
"Variations in the Incidence of Surgery." *New England Journal of Medicine* 281:880–884.

Luft, H.
1978
"How Do Health Maintenance Organizations Achieve Their 'Savings': Rhetoric and Evidence." *New England Journal of Medicine* 298:1336–43.

Luft, H., et al.
1979
"Should Operations Be Regionalized? The Empirical Relation between Surgical Volume and Mortality." *New England Journal of Medicine* 301:1364–69.

Martin, L.
1972
"Cost and Management of Intensive Care." *Modern Hospital* 118:97–99.

McCarthy, E., and G. Widmer
1974
"Effects of Screening by Consultants on Recommended Elective Surgical Procedures." *New England Journal of Medicine* 291:1331–35.

McClure, W.
1976
"Reducing Excess Hospital Capacity." Excelsior, Minn.: Interstudy, October 15.

McMahon, J. A.
1979
Statement on Behalf of the American Hospital Association during Hearings before the Subcommittee on Health of the Committee on Finance, on Health Cost Containment. U.S. Senate, 96th Congress. March 13, 14.

Mitchell, B. M., and C. E. Phelps
1976
"National Health Insurance: Some Costs and Effects of Mandated Employee Coverage." *Journal of Political Economy* 84:553–572.

Moore, F.
1978
"What to Do When Physicians Disagree: A Second Look at Second Opinions." *Archives of Surgery* 113:1397–1400.

Morton, J., et al.
1968
"Evaluation of Surgical Bed Utilization." *Archives of Surgery* 97:395.

National Academy of Sciences
1979
Medical Technology and the Health Care System: A Study of the Diffusion of Equipment Embodied Technology. Committee on Technology and Health Care of the National Research Council and the Institute of Medicine. Washington, D.C.

New York Medical Society
1970
Report of the Cholecystectomy Subcommittee of the Quality of Care Committee.

New York Medical Society
1972
Report of the Hysterectomy Subcommittee of the Quality of Care Committee.

Newhouse, J. P.
1970
"Toward a Theory of Non-Profit Institutions: An Economic Model of a Hospital." *American Economic Review* 60:145–155.

Newhouse, J. P.
1974
Forecasting the Demand for Medical Care for the Purposes of Planning Health Services. Santa Monica, Cal.: Rand Corporation, R-1635-OEO.

Newhouse, J. P.
1978
The Economics of Medical Care. Reading, Mass.: Addison-Wesley.

Newhouse, J. P., and V. Taylor
1971
"How Shall We Pay for Hospital Care?" *Public Interest.* Spring.

Office of Technology Assessment
1978
Assessing the Efficacy and Safety of Medical Technologies. Washington, D.C.

Office of Technology Assessment
1978
Policy Implications of the Computed Tomographic Scanner. Washington, D.C.

Pauly, M.
1979
"Overinsurance: The Conceptual Issues." Mimeographed.

Pauly, M., and M. Redisch
1973
"The Not-for-Profit Hospital as a Physicians' Cooperative." *American Economic Review* 63:87–100.

Peltzman, S.
1973
"An Evaluation of Consumer Protection Legislation: The 1962 Drug Amendments." *Journal of Political Economy* 81:1049–91.

Policy Analysis, Inc.
1980
Evaluation of the Effects of Certificate-of-Need Programs, vol. 3, Draft Final Report. (With Urban Systems Research and Engineering Inc.)

Posner, R.
1974
"Certificate-of-Need for Health Care Facilities: A Dissenting View." In

C. Havighurst, ed., *Regulating Health Facilities Construction*. Washington, D.C.: American Enterprise Institute.

Rabkin, M. T., and C. N. Melin
1978
"The Impact of Technology upon the Cost and Quality of Hospital Care and a Proposal for Control of New and Expensive Technology." In R. Egdahl and P. Gertman, eds., *Technology and the Quality of Health Care*. Germantown: Aspen Systems Corporation.

Rapoport, J.
1978
"Diffusion of Technological Innovation among Nonprofit Firms: A Case Study of Radioisotopes in U.S. Hospitals." *Journal of Economics and Business* 30:108–118.

Roemer, M. I., and M. Shain
1959
"Hospital Utilization under Insurance." Chicago: American Hospital Association.

Russell, L.
1979
Technology in Hospitals. Washington, D.C.: Brookings.

Rutkow, I. M., and G. D. Zuidema
1978
" 'Unnecessary Surgery': An Update." *Surgery* 63:671–678.

Salkever, D. C., and T. W. Bice
1976
"The Impact of Certificate-of-Need Controls on Hospital Investment." *Milbank Memorial Fund Quarterly* 54:185–214.

Sattler, F., ed.
1976
Hospital Prospective Payment: Issues and Experiences. Minneapolis, Minn.: Interstudy.

Schwartz, W., and P. L. Joskow
1980a
"Duplicated Hospital Facilities." *New England Journal of Medicine* 303:1449–57.

Schwartz, W. and P. Joskow
1980b
"The Medical and Economic Implications of Disagreement between Surgeons—A Reappraisal of the Second Opinion." Mimeographed.

Schwartz, W. and P. Joskow
1978
"Medical Efficacy versus Economic Efficiency: A Conflict in Values." *New England Journal of Medicine* 299:1462–64.

Shain, M., and R. Roemer
1959
"Hospital Costs Relate to the Supply of Beds." *Modern Hospital* 92(4):71–73.

Sheshinski, E.
1971
"Welfare Aspects of a Regulatory Constraint: Note." *American Economic Review* 61:175–178.

Sloan, F. A., and B. Steinwald
1980
"Effects of Regulation on Hospital Costs and Input Use." *Journal of Law and Economics* 23(1):81–110.

Spence, A. M.
1976
"Product Selection, Fixed Costs, and Monopolistic Competition." *Review of Economic Studies* 43:217–235.

Stuart, B. C.
1976
"Medicaid Cost Containment Policy: Utilization Controls." The Urban Institute, Working Paper No. 986-08.

Trussell, R. E., et al.
1962
"The Quantity, Quality, and Costs of Medical and Hospital Care Secured by a Sample of Teamster Families in the New York Area." Columbia University School of Public Health and Administrative Medicine.

U.S. Congress
1974
Senate Subcommittee on Antitrust and Monopoly of the Committee on the Judiciary. Hearings: *Competition in the Health Services Market*, parts 1–3, 93rd Congress, May and July, 1974. Washington, D.C.

U.S. Department of Health, Education and Welfare
1975
Bureau of Health Planning and Resources Development. "Health Care Facilities: Existing and Needed. Hill-Burton State Plan Data as of January, 1975.

Warner, K. E.
1979
"The Cost of Capital-Embodied Medical Technology." In National Academy of Sciences, *Medical Technology and the Health Care System*.

Wagner, J. L., and M. Zubkoff
1978
"Medical Technology and Hospital Costs." In M. Zubkoff et al., eds., *Hospital Cost Containment: Selected Notes for Future Policy*. New York: Prodist.

Weiner, S. M.
1977
" 'Reasonable Cost' Reimbursement for Inpatient Hospital Services under Medicare and Medicaid: The Emergence of Public Control." *American Journal of Law and Medicine* 3:1–47.

Weinstein, R., and J. DeMarco
1979
"Prospective Ratesetting in Massachusetts." *Topics in Health Care Financing* 6:69–80.

Wennberg, J.
1975
"Getting Ready for National Health Insurance: Unnecessary Surgery." Testimony and Statement presented at Hearings before the Subcommittee on Oversight and Investigations of the Committee on Interstate and Foreign Commerce, House of Representatives, 94th Congress (No. 94-37), July 15.

Wennberg, J., and A. Gittelsohn
1975
"Health Care Delivery in Maine, I: Patterns of Use of Common Surgical Procedures." *Journal of the Maine Medical Association* 46:123–149.

Wennberg, J.
1973
"Small-Area Variations in Health Care." *Science* 182:1102–1108.

Worthington, N. L., K. Tyson, and M. Chin
1979
"Prospective Reimbursement in Maryland." *Topics in Health Care Financing* 6:60–68.

Wortzman, G., et al.
1975
"Cranial Computed Tomography: An Evaluation of Cost Effectiveness." *Radiology* 117:75–77.

Zeckhauser, R.
1979
"Using the Wrong Tool: The Pursuit of Redistribution through Regulation." Mimeographed.

Zeckhauser, R.
1970
"Medical Insurance: A Case Study of the Tradeoff between Risk Spreading and Appropriate Incentives." *Journal of Economic Theory* 2:10–26.

Index